ADVANCE PRAISE FOR

Vodka Is Vegan

And The Vegan Bros

"The Vegan Bros kick a**! Their new book educates and enlightens in a fun way, showing that eating vegan is for people from all walks of life. I recommend it to anyone thinking about making the switch!"
—DANIELLA MONET, actress and activist

"*Vodka Is Vegan* makes the case for a vegan diet in a way that's both hilarious and non-judgmental. The Vegan Bros recognize that everyone is on their own unique path and encourage you on every step you take."   —NATHAN RUNKLE, founder of Mercy For Animals

"Do you know how many NFL players are switching over to plant-based diets? I see it all the time! Look no further than the very best, Tom Brady. But it's not just a 5x Super Bowl champ that understands the benefits. *Vodka Is Vegan* is humorous, inspiring, and, most important, educational on WHY the world is choosing to go VEGAN!"
—ERIN COSCARELLI,
sportscaster and TV host, NFL Network

"If you think going vegan is a great idea, but not for "regular" people like you, think again. The Vegan Bros hilarious and insightful new book shows you the way to a healthier, happier, cruelty-free, new you. A fast, funny, and life-changing read!"
—SUZY WELCH, bestselling author

"Hilarious and informative. *Vodka Is Vegan* is one of the funniest books I've read. If you like dogs and don't want to eat them then this book is for you."   —CRAIG COCHRAN,
cofounder of Terri restaurant and P.S. Kitchen

"*Vodka Is Vegan* is an absolute ice breaker to get everyone talking about veganism. The Vegan Bros obliterate stereotypes and make their case for vegan world domination in a charming way that will tear down walls. A much-needed book!" —FLORIAN RADKE, cofounder of Cinnaholic and marketing guru

"Having long been associated with sprawling, armpit-hair-clad, animal-rights warrior types, the animal-product-free lifestyle is now more closely aligned with ripped, mildly hipster-ish gym bunnies such as bolshy bloggers Vegan Bros." —*Vice*

"If you want to see the face—or, to be more accurate, the body—of the new wave of veganism, head to the website of the Vegan Bros." —*The Guardian* (London)

"When speaking with them, it is hard not to think: If this lacrosse-room ebullience is the product of a plant-based diet, I want in." —*Grist*

VODKA IS VEGAN

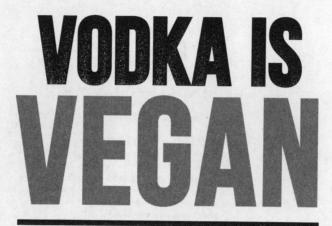

VODKA IS VEGAN

A MANIFESTO
FOR BETTER LIVING
AND NOT BEING AN A**HOLE

PHIL & MATT LETTEN
THE VEGAN BROS

A TarcherPerigee Book

tarcherperigee

An imprint of Penguin Random House LLC
375 Hudson Street
New York, New York 10014

Most TarcherPerigee books are available at special quantity discounts for bulk purchase for sales promotions, premiums, fund-raising, and educational needs. Special books or book excerpts also can be created to fit specific needs. For details, write: SpecialMarkets@penguinrandomhouse.com.

Library of Congress Cataloging-in-Publication Data
Names: Letten, Matt, author. | Letten, Phil, author.
Title: Vodka is vegan : a Vegan Bros manifesto for better living and not being an a**hole / Matt Letten, Phil Letten, the Vegan Bros.
Description: New York, New York : A TarcherPerigee Book, 2018. | Includes bibliographical references. |
Identifiers: LCCN 2018009209 (print) | LCCN 2018012641 (ebook) | ISBN 9781101993378 (e-book) | ISBN 9780143129738 (paperback)
Subjects: LCSH: Veganism. | Animal welfare. | BISAC: HEALTH & FITNESS / Healthy Living. | SELF-HELP / General.
Classification: LCC TX392 (ebook) | LCC TX392 .L4927 2018 (print) | DDC 613.2/622—dc23
LC record available at https://lccn.loc.gov/2018009209

Printed in the United States of America
1 3 5 7 9 10 8 6 4 2

To our parents.

Mom, let's be honest, you're probably the only reason either of us actually graduated from high school. You hustled us from church to soccer, to baseball, to basketball, and you probably single-handedly wrote most of our meaningful reports in school. We always knew we were the most important things in your life.

Dad, your day job as a commercial pilot had you traveling nonstop, but somehow you managed to be our best friend, our coach, and our biggest cheerleader. You instilled in us the idea that somehow we could accomplish anything we wanted. And here we are having written an actual book.

Lillie, Skyler, and Peyton. You showed us the emotional bond and connection we are capable of having with animals. The joy you all had for playing ball and taking rides in the car was contagious. You are the reason we fight for all animals.

Set your mind on a definite goal and

observe how quickly the world

stands aside to let you pass.

—NAPOLEON HILL

CONTENTS

INTRODUCTION

Hi—WE'RE PHIL AND MATT. We're brothers. We're writers. And we're vegan.

First off, you might ask, "Are you guys also pieces of shit?"

No. There is a difference between "vegan" and "piece of shit." But there are the people who are both at the same time.

We, on the other hand, do our best to have love for everyone. And we know you may have interacted with a "vegan piece of shit" in the past. On behalf of all the vegans and all the animals, we're sorry you experienced that.

We totally understand if you want to let that experience, or those experiences, cloud the way you view vegan eating. But we beg you to give us another chance.

If Beyoncé, Jay-Z, Jared Leto, Mike Tyson, Kylie Jenner, Serena Williams, Miley Cyrus, Liam Hemsworth, Olivia Wilde, Tony Gonzalez, Joaquin Phoenix, and Brad Pitt are exploring it or 100 percent on-board now, then maybe we're on to something with this whole "vegan" thing.

A vegan is two things:

1) Someone who thinks it's wrong to brutally torture and kill animals. That's 90 percent of the definition.
2) Someone who doesn't support torturing animals with their diet. That's the last 10 percent that most of us have fucked up on.

We acknowledge that we're all on our own unique personal journey. Rather than look for ways to exclude people, we try to be as inclusive as possible. If you're opposed to animal abuse and you enjoy fruit or, hell, an Oreo (yes, they're vegan), guess what? You're already 90 percent vegan. We're just here to help you get that final 10 percent. Or at least move a few more percentage points up.

One of the reasons that we wanted to write this book was because, as veganism has risen and become very popular in the mainstream, there was also a small segment of vegans who were assholes.

There used to be a joke about vegans. "A vegan walks into a bar . . . and I only know this because he told everyone within two minutes." Okay, we get it. Vegans were pretty outspoken about their veganity in the past.

But it's not that way anymore.

We became vegans for two basic reasons: we loved animals, and we wanted to be healthy and fit. Refusing to eat animals, and products derived from animals, helps spare a bunch of adorable critters torture and death while also keeping us toned as fuck. And that's good. But we also want people to know what eating vegan is NOT.

Eating vegan is NOT . . .

1. A way for you to feel superior to other people. Hey, we're all human, we're all composed of similar weaknesses and flaws. And for a lot of people, one big commonality is that we want to matter, we want to stand out, we want to be special. A productive way to achieve that perfectly reasonable goal is to do things like learn shit, work out, and have stimulating conversations with interesting people and *listen* to what they have to say. A less productive way to achieve this goal is to try to put people down. And a lot of people have done this. Instead of saying something interesting, they would just shit all over what someone else said. Instead of helping someone and being awesome, they would rag on someone for being selfish. And that's how some vegans gave the word "vegan" a bad rep. They adopted

a super-aggro vegan stance purely as a way to make other people feel shitty and make themselves seem, by contrast, superior. That's some bullshit right there. We don't believe in that negative shit. We're all about positivity! We want people to eat vegan because of the amazing, compelling reasons to eat vegan, and not because we'll label them as pieces of shit if they don't.

2. Some kind of higher plane of existence. Eating vegan is *how you eat*. This is, we think, what used to drive away a lot of people from eating vegan. They thought it was some weird cult that had lots of rules, and if you broke those rules by eating a brownie made with butter, then you would be banished from the society forever, condemned for the rest of time to feel like a failure and an outsider. And that shit's just not so. Being vegan isn't like being part of Opus Dei or the Promise Keepers or Heaven's Gate. Eating vegan doesn't mean you can't associate with meat-eating friends. It doesn't mean you have to wear fur, leather, etc. or only go to vegan-only restaurants or coffeehouses. And it sure as shit doesn't mean that if you eat a veggie burger made on the same grill as a beef burger that you get sent to vegan prison or vegan hell or are publicly disconnected in some humiliating ceremony. Eating vegan just means you prefer to not eat food made from animals. Let's keep the pressure low.

We also wanted to write this book as a way to address something we saw as an important cultural progression. We're bros. Literally, we're brothers, but we're also a couple of guys who like to party, and for lots of people, it's incomprehensible that we're also vegan. They have this image of vegans as these crunchy hippies who just spend the day in a drum circle, or as pencil-necked hipsters who play in ironic kickball leagues and vape aerosolized patchouli (also ironically). And as far as that goes, we honestly don't think there's anything wrong with it.

But it's also just not the way it is. Vegans can also be bros who love to party. They can be artists with nothing but contempt for the czars of fashion. They can be ballerinas or linebackers. They can be lawyers, doctors, construction workers, accountants, Beatles fans, Elvis fans, Veronica lovers, Betty lovers, Prius drivers, and pickup truck drivers. It's everyone. It's all of us. It's inclusive. You don't have to be part of a certain group to eat vegan, and you don't have to change anything about yourself to become a vegan (other than not eating animals). This is a big tent. Everyone is welcome.

We hope to see you inside.

CHAPTER 1

EARLY DAYS: PORTRAIT OF TWO FUTURE VEGANS AS MEAT LOVERS

WE DON'T EAT MEAT. And that's because we hate it, we've always hated it, we find it repulsive, and we've only ever eaten tofu all our lives. Right?

Wrong.

We weren't born by springing out of a pod and then munching on the grass. We're a couple of normal, red-blooded American guys who grew up like a lot of other guys. We used to eat meat. We used to *love* eating meat. For breakfast, we'd eat bacon with a fucking side of sausage. Our club sandwich was a layer of turkey, a layer of bacon, a layer of ham, and some lettuce as a garnish. Probably with a side of bacon. Dinner was a turducken. So we loved meat.

But meat didn't always love us back.

This asymmetry became obvious to us when we were still very young, about seven and ten years old, when we went on vacation in Puerto Rico.

The trip was awesome. Our dad had been a captain for Delta, so we got to take lots of free flights. It was both a vacation and an anniversary present for our grandparents, who joined us on the trip. It was our very first vacation to a tropical island, and we discovered that we fucking *love* tropical islands. What's not to love? It's warm, there's a nice breeze, pineapples grow out of the ground as if by magic, you can swim in the ocean, and everyone seems really nice and in a great mood (perhaps caused by all the warm weather and the pineapples and the beaches).

And we weren't one of those families that checks in at the hotel and then just hangs out by the pool all day and eats in the hotel restaurant at night, and then lather, rinse, repeat for a week. We liked doing shit. We stayed at a coffee plantation in the mountains (possibly where we started a fascination with the bean that would culminate in our becoming full-fledged coffee nerds), we saw a castle in Old San Juan, and we saw plenty of beaches.

FUN FACT: Americans consume a shitload of coffee, to the tune of about 400 million cups per day and 146 billion cups per year. We drink most of ours at Starbucks.

And when we were there, we didn't just tan, we did shit, like snorkeling, kayaking, exploring a side island overrun with iguanas (Iguana Island), and making our first attempts at surfing. The results perhaps explain why you're not reading a surfing manifesto.

We even went to church. Our family had a policy that when we went on vacation, there was still no vacation from church. God didn't take days off, dude. And our dad would want to go to places that were really part of the culture of the places we'd be visiting. So we went to this tiny Spanish-speaking church, where a guy who spoke English tried to serve as an interpreter (even though our dad spoke Spanish), and later we visited a Puerto Rican megachurch. It was an experience! The reverend spoke with a microphone and sound system (the most efficient way to reach a few thousand parishioners), they did laying on of hands, the whole nine yards. People were excited to share their faith with us, and we were super jazzed about experiencing Puerto Rican culture.

It was a blast!

But things went south when we tried to make them a bit meatier.

McD, POR FAVOR

Our family saw this trip as an opportunity to sample the local culture. And one of the most pleasurable ways to do that was through the food. There were *mallorcas* (ham and cheese sandwiches). There was *chillo frito* (fried red snapper). There was *sancocho* (chicken and root vegetable soup). There were *almojábanas* (cheese fritters). There was ramp *escabeche* (ramps grilled in garlic). There was *conquito* French toast (French toast with an amazing coconut flavor). There was *arroz con gandules* (rice with pigeon peas). There was *mofongo con salsa de tomate* (mashed plantains with tomato sauce). There were *tostones* (fried plantains). Suffice it to say, there was a lot of different stuff to eat.

Unless you were Phil.

There we were, sitting around a table at a nice restaurant in San Juan, looking at menus and trying to figure out what to eat.

"I'm thinking of the *bacalao*, this fish stew thing," said our dad.

"I think I'll have the *tostones* and maybe the rice and beans," our mom said.

"I'm going to have the octopus," Matt said.

"Really? That seems adventurous," said our dad.

"Well, an octopus bit me yesterday, so this is how I get my revenge," Matt said. "What about you, Phil?"

"This looks gross," Phil said, pushing away his menu like it was a colony of maggots.

"That's not true," said our mom. "There are plenty of delicious things on the menu. You just haven't tried them before."

"Seafood is disgusting. I want a burger."

"I don't think there are any burgers on the menu," our dad said.

"Then let's go to a place that does have burgers on the menu," Phil replied. "I think I saw a McDonald's down the road. Let's go there."

"We're eating here," our dad said.

"Damn you, old man! You may be able to land a 747 on a mosquito's butthole, but you're not getting me to do shit! Now get me a Big Mac!"

Okay, seven-year-old Phil didn't actually drop a ton of F-bombs at dinner, but he sure as hell threw a fit. He did NOT want to eat Puerto Rican food. So he bitched and he moaned and eventually got our mom to agree to a stop at the Golden Arches after our regular dinner. Moms are funny that way. You threaten to starve a child, even if it's the child who's threatening the starvation, and the moms will fold faster than Superman on laundry day. No *sofrito* for Phil.

So we had a delicious dinner of plantains and beans and rice and some octopus and cod, and then we went to McDonald's and got Phil his Quarter Pounder with cheese and some fries. And, of course, Matt, who was large and in charge, couldn't quite resist. If we were getting something for Phil, then it would be wrong to deny getting Matt something as well, so he'd follow up on his dinner with a second dinner of McDonald's. A cheeseburger or two is the traditional *digestif* after a nice octopus; any gourmand will tell you that.

The whole thing was one big shame detour. Our grandparents had lived during the Great Depression, so they just couldn't understand why Phil would refuse to eat perfectly good food so that he could be served a hamburger of questionable quality. Our parents wouldn't even go inside the restaurant. We'd get the food through the drive-in, so nobody could see us and so the Puerto Rican locals wouldn't witness us being the stereotype of Americans who come to another place and then refuse to eat anything other than McDonald's or Burger King or KFC. Then we'd drive off as fast as we could while Phil stuffed himself with his whiner's booty.

You'd think that there would have been enough factors to give Phil a greater appreciation for the food he was being offered. When we were on Iguana Island, our guide also showed us an area full of what looked like nightmare boats. Calling them boats at all was pretty charitable, because these shitty rafts were little more than a few wooden planks and good intentions. They'd come to the island from Cuba, full of refugees looking for a better life. These boats must have been scary as fuck to sail from Cuba to Puerto Rico. But that's exactly what these refugees did. They took a chance. And they made it. Though we knew we couldn't see the ones that had gone to the bottom. But those people would have been happy to get some rice and beans, and here was Phil turning his nose up at it. How was that possible?

Maybe it wasn't so unlikely that Phil would have become enthralled and obsessed with something that wasn't necessarily in his best interests. Back then, that seemed to be just part of his personality. He showed the same kind of behavior when we visited the casino in our hotel. Phil LOVED the casino. Was this because Phil was an absolute shark at baccarat and paid for our entire vacation with his winnings? No. Was this because Phil got his vodka cranberries comped while he was at the gaming tables? No—Phil only drank Long Island iced teas as a seven-year-old. Was this because Phil was inspired by the singers and comedians working the stage, dreaming of a career as an entertainer? Not quite. Mostly, Phil loved the blinking lights. He loved the electronic displays of the slot machines. Both Phil and Matt loved video games, and the casino looked like an entire building devoted to video games! You pushed in a quarter, lights would blink, bells and whistles and beeps and growls would sound, and sometimes, money would come out. Phil loved all of that. Maybe there was just something about Phil's brain at seven that was starved for a kind of instant stimulation. And slot machines and McDonald's cheeseburgers both seemed to scratch that itch for him.

It was kind of amazing. Here we were, a family trying to enjoy Puerto Rican culture and one another's company, and that all gets destroyed because Phil insists on going to a "family" restaurant! And it would happen every night. Every night! Our parents would try to find a nice little spot to eat, and Phil would flip his shit about how he needed some cheeseburgers from McDonald's, and our mom would try to avoid an intranational incident and calm his ass down, and we'd hit the drive-through.

So that was the low point.

But it wasn't the only one.

Another big part of the vacation was going fishing.

WE'RE ON A BOAT!

Our grandpa must have been Quint or Ahab in a past life (even though both those guys were fictional characters, but referencing a great historical fisherman is kind of useless, so here we are), because he LOVED fishing. And so we looked forward to it, too. And on this trip, since it was partly an anniversary present for him, we had a special treat: a deep-sea-fishing charter.

This wasn't the kind of fishing where you slip on hip waders and stand knee-deep in a river and think about the sun rising and paint watercolor landscapes in your mind. This was the "bring it on" kind of fishing. This was the type of fishing like in *Jaws*, where you strap yourself into a chair that's bolted to the deck, because the kinds of fish that you're hunting for are hundreds of pounds and would rip you right out of the boat if you snagged them without some kind of anchor. With these rigs, you could go after swordfish or marlin.

We were fishing for mahi-mahi in Puerto Rico. Now, mahi-mahi aren't as big as marlin, but they can top off at about forty pounds, which is about the size of a four-year-old child. And if you hooked into some preschooler on a fishing boat, it would pull the rod out of your hands if you weren't anchored in. And then you'd go to jail, because it's illegal in Puerto Rico to fish for children (but not in Florida, which was a surprise to us all).

Keep in mind that we didn't quite understand how fishing worked. We knew that you put bait on a hook, and put the hook in the water, but then the details kind of got fuzzy for us. We just assumed that you'd hook a fish in the mouth, he would instantly die in a pretty painless way, then you haul him into the boat, and upon making contact with the deck, he'd just kind of disassemble into a bunch of filets.

Not quite.

When you hook a fish, sometimes you get her in the mouth. Sometimes you don't. Sometimes you hook her in her eye. That's a horrible thing to see, pulling a fish the size of a child up by her eyeball. Sometimes the fish gets the bait and swallows it, which means that when you pull on the rod, it doesn't pull on the tough skin of the fish's mouth (which is also pretty horrible when you think about it), but is instead pulling on the soft organs. Sometimes, that just rips her stomach right out, which seems a fucking awful way to die.

Usually, however, the hook will catch in a fish's mouth. Then you battle it for a while, reel her in, and haul her onto the boat. That's the best-case scenario. And even then, it was pretty terrible to watch. Our grandpa wasn't just pulling a fish onto the deck of the boat and then giving her a lethal injection. He was reeling her in as far as he could, and then someone on the boat would "help" the fish by trapping her with a gaffing hook. This is a pretty medieval-looking implement, and it's not some catcher's mitt that handles the fish into the boat, it's a metal hook that rips into the mahi-mahi's side to gain control over it. Blood spurts everywhere, because you're basically stabbing a fish to death. Then you get her on board and smash her in the head with a club. Now you can eat her!

Whoa, whoa, whoa, whoa! It is not, at this point, ready to eat. First you have to *clean* her. And we can't envision a more misleading term than "cleaning" a fish, because there's nothing clean about it. When you really get down to it, it's actually pretty weird and disgusting. This is when you rip out the guts and throw them in the chum bucket for future trips. We couldn't really participate in the cleaning process. That was for the adults, because we sure as hell didn't want to have a hand in that. That, perhaps, should have been a clue to us. If part of the preparation for a meal involves something so gross or so offensive or so sickening that you can't do it *or even watch it*, then maybe that is the sort of thing you shouldn't be eating to begin with. "Yeah, I'll have those hummingbird wings for you in a second. First, I just have to remove them with a pair of rusty pliers and then stick some bamboo shoots under its toenails for kicks and then pour some turpentine on it." Yeah, I'll pass.

But we ate it that night. Except for Phil, who insisted on going to the fucking McDonald's.

Knowing where that food came from definitely altered our interest in eating it. And that's something that most people never experience. If you do all your shopping in a supermarket, all you see are pristine, bloodless fillets of fish, perfectly butchered steaks, chickens with no beaks or eyes. The food doesn't even look like an animal, really, which is intentional. If people had to fish for their own mahi-mahi, if they had to hunt for their own pork chops, they might realize the pain and the cost involved in acquiring those proteins, and maybe they would make the switch to something better.

We didn't become vegetarians that day, but that trip laid some of the groundwork. We learned what kind of pain a fish goes through before she becomes a meal. (This gal had it pretty good though compared to a lot of her fish friends that are destined to a life of underwater imprisonment in small tanks crammed with thousands upon thousands of fish.) We learned what kind of deprivation a refugee faces. And most important, we learned that the only people who insist on a McDonald's hamburger, when there are plenty of delicious and healthier options available, are probably folks who just don't know any better. Phil was just seven and had some time to figure his shit out, and if you're reading this, we hope you're coming to the same conclusion that he did, a conclusion he'd arrive at only a few years down the line. . . .

CHAPTER 2

PHIL DECIDES TO STOP BEING A MASSIVE PILE OF SHIT, OR PHIL'S LIFE TRANSFORMATION

I DON'T EAT MEAT, or products made from meat. And you know how that came to be? It sure wasn't because my family was vegan and that's just how I grew up, because my mom and dad were farrrrrrrrr from the vegan types.

My dad was a pilot. You know who else was a pilot? Chuck Yeager. The dude once shot down five enemy planes in a single day—he became an ace in one day! And Yeager wasn't just a pilot, he was a test pilot, which is like the difference between a kid who plays Pop-A-Shot and an NBA All-Star. Chuck Yeager did amazing things in the air. When the military unveiled a new plane, they said, "Hey, Chuck—take this one up and let us know how everything holds together." Sometimes that would mean that the cockpit glass would ice up at ten thousand feet and he'd get frostbite on his fingers chipping it off. Or he'd have to set the plane down with no landing gear. And here's another little footnote on his résumé: he broke the sound barrier. The first man to travel faster than the speed of sound! And you know what he got for that performance?

According to *The Right Stuff*, he got a free steak, and all the trimmings, at Pancho's Happy Bottom Riding Club.

That's right. The reward for breaking *the motherfucking sound barrier* was a cut of beef. So guess what we ate with great appreciation in our house: meat.

That's how I was raised. Maybe kind of clueless and insulated and more than a little entitled (as illustrated by my time in Puerto Rico rejecting delicious fried plantains in order to get fucking McDonald's). But then I saw some shit that I could not easily unsee, amigos, and it fucked with my head pretty good until I realized I had to do something about it.

HOLY SHIT . . . A WAKE-UP CALL

It was fall of my senior year in high school in 2004, and like most kids in the fall of their senior years, I was at a concert. I'd come to see Most Precious Blood, a hard-core band that was playing in the Shelter, the basement venue of St. Andrews Hall in Detroit. I was sporting a

Mohawk, a thrift-store jacket, and about fifteen bracelets up my arm, including a couple of necklaces and a decapitated dress sock.

It wasn't just some standard show. Most Precious Blood was music with a conscience. Or at least musicians with something on their minds. They held strong political and ethical beliefs. These beliefs were so strong, in fact, that in between songs they invited a guy up onstage to drop some truth bombs on the crowd.

"My friend Johnny got fucking arrested last night! And what did he do? Did he rob a goddamn liquor store? Did he shoot a cop? Did he set a house on fire? Hell no, he didn't! He set some animals free! Went up to a fur farm, jumped the fence, and he set a couple of dozen minks free! And they arrested him for it! Can you believe it? They arrested him because he didn't want some asshole to kill a defenseless animal so that some rich lady in New York could wear a goddamn fur coat so she wouldn't get cold walking from the lobby of her fancy apartment building to the cab waiting on the street! Does that sound like justice to you?"

Hell no, that didn't sound like justice. That sounded like a horror show. And not like the horror of *28 Days Later*, which starts with a bunch of activists trying to set animals free from a lab, which leads directly to the release of the Rage Virus and the beginning of the zombie apocalypse. That was an awesome movie. This fur farm didn't sound so awesome. So I thought it was pretty cool, this band that I had come to see letting this guy take the stage to talk about his friend who got arrested. He said he had some literature in the back, and I thought that was cool, too. A lot of the time, you check out a show, and if there's any kind of merch, it's the band's CD or a T-shirt or some shit like that. These guys put out a table with *literature*? Okay, you got my attention.

So I go to the back of the Shelter, and a colored piece of paper with cows on the cover caught my eye. *Now, that's an unusual piece of pornography*, I thought, and had to investigate. But it wasn't anything sordid—it was a twelve-page pamphlet explaining everything about the meat industry, and I read that shit from cover to cover.

Imagine you're Chuck Yeager in his X-1, cruising along at about forty-five thousand feet, just having a great day. You're about to break the sound barrier, the sun is shining, not a cloud in the sky, birds are singing . . . and then you smash into one at 770 mph.

What.

The . . .

?!

I couldn't believe what I read. Just like Yeager smashing into a bird at the speed of sound, this was horrible, bloody, and it made quite an impression. Here's some of the knowledge that got dropped on my seventeen-year-old head that day.

PLIERS ARE NOT MEDICAL EQUIPMENT

For most factory farms, pigs aren't kept in the big, roomy, friendly pens shown in *Babe* or *Charlotte's Web* or even *Animal Farm* (which is not a happy story at all, but the depiction of the conditions that the pigs live in sure seems a lot more luxurious). As I saw in the photo in the pamphlet, most pigs were confined to crates barely bigger than their own bodies. Can you imagine a person being forced to be in a room, a closet, so small that they can't even turn around? Or lie down? That would be a goddamn war crime. I wanted to stop reading, but I kept going.

> **WTF:** A gestation crate typically measures only *2 feet wide.* Basically, it's really, really small.

Soon I learned that there wasn't one single federal law that protects farm animals from abuse. And this shit was standard practice in the pork industry. It wasn't like this photo was from the only farm in the world that did this. And it wasn't Photoshopped. This shit was real.

And it only got worse.

Testosterone can make a pig more aggressive, and it can also adversely affect the flavor of the meat when hormones are released during the terror of slaughter. So you know what the pork industry does as a solution to this problem? They just rip the testicles off conscious piglets without any kind of anesthetic or surgical training. Just rip their junk right the fuck off. And sometimes, crazy as it sounds, this procedure, done by poorly paid and poorly trained workers, doesn't always work perfectly. Often, piglets will suffer from herniated intestines because of their barbaric method of castration.

So the pork industry doesn't think it's a good idea for pigs to have their balls. You know what other parts they don't think that pigs require? Their tails. Pig tails are dumb. Who the fuck needs 'em? They can get damaged or eaten by neighboring pigs, which can lead to infection and revenue loss. Some might see that problem and propose, as a solution, "Maybe these pigs need more space so that their tails aren't always up against other pigs' mouths!" Not the pork industry. Nope, the pork industry's solution is to just grab a pair of dull clippers, get ahold of that tail in their rusty teeth, and just rip it right off.

You know what else they rip off? Teeth. Baby pigs can be quite determined to get to their mother for suckling, and sometimes they bite. The pork industry has a solution for this problem: they rip their teeth out. Because who needs teeth anyway, right? Sometimes they pull the teeth, and sometimes they grind them down with some kind of abrasive tool. Can you imagine this as a solution to your biting issues? "Hey, dentist, I'm grinding my teeth in my sleep. What do you think—maybe a mouth guard?" "Hell no—let me get my industrial grinder and sand those suckers down.

Problem solved!" Whoever does this job probably thinks the movie *Marathon Man* is hilarious. I immediately regret inserting this movie reference. My hands are covering my mouth and I feel like my mouth is about to be stabbed.

What if a pig gets sick or hurt? Which can happen all too easily from infections developed from improper castration or tail removal or agonizing pressure sores. Many of those pigs just get shoved to the side and allowed to suffer until they die. Would a person allow a dog or a cat to die this way? Maybe if they had a good reason, like the dog or cat stole their husband or wife away or burned their house to the ground or changed their Netflix password without telling anyone, but otherwise, no, of course that wouldn't be fucking okay. So why is it okay to do it to a pig and not another animal? Intelligence? Hell, pigs are smarter than dogs. It's why they took over in *Animal Farm*. Fucking Napoleon. Snowball should have been running that show.

The pork industry openly admitted that this was how they did business. As I turned the pages on the pamphlet I'd picked up, I learned that shit was similar for chickens as well.

DO CHICKENS LIKE BEING ABUSED?

Chickens have no teeth to rip out, so they're on easy street, right? Wrong-o. Hens are confined inside tiny cages called battery cages. A battery cage is a tiny wire cage that confines

19

about five birds. The cages are stacked on top of one another, so the hens are shitting all over one another. And we know what your first question is: "Are the birds given enough space to at least spread their wings?" And the answer is, "No, you asshole! What kind of monster wants to allow an intelligent animal enough space to spread her wings? You're sick!"

> **WTF:** The battery cages that chickens are confined to measure about 67 square inches. A standard piece of paper is 93.5 square inches. So there's about 50 percent more space on a piece of paper you'd find in a copier at Kinko's compared to a battery cage.

Being in such close quarters means that these birds naturally peck at each other, and a pecked-over bird doesn't seem as appetizing, so what do the chicken farmers do? They cut their beaks off with a red-hot blade is what they do. This is done without the benefit of painkillers, and the debeaking machinery often goes too far and cuts into their faces. But, I mean, big deal, right?

And that's just the hens. How about the male chicks? Well, the male chicks don't produce eggs, so they're not as useful. Typically, male chicks are either ground up while still living, gassed to death, or suffocated. Then they take the bits of chicken that are ground up and turn it into things like dog food or fertilizer.

Though at least those chicks are spared what happens to

broiler chickens. Those chickens, prized for their meat, are fed massive amounts of shit to get their weight up. Imagine a two-year-old toddler that's somehow force-fed to the point that it tips the scales at 350 pounds and you'll have some idea of how unnatural this is. This makes the birds suffer from health defects and many are unable to walk, unable to support their giant body at such a young age. And many suffer heart attacks.

This is what happens to these animals. I couldn't believe it.

It was one of those WTF moments.

When I got home from the concert, I told my parents about what I'd learned.

"Mom, Dad, I think the meat industry might be evil."

"If you're upset about the McRib, I don't even think that counts as meat," my dad said.

"No, I mean the things they do to animals—it's just insane."

"Circle of life," my mom said, then broke into the song from *The Lion King*. Her choreography was amazing.

"But it's just so cruel!" I described what I'd read in the pamphlet.

"I think that's just propaganda that the activist groups put out there," my mom said. "I mean, sure, I'm not naïve, and I'll bet there are some bad apples who do things like you describe, but those are just a few farms. That's not how they do it in most places."

I nodded, because I wanted to believe them. I wanted to think it was true that what I'd seen applied to only a small percentage of the animals in the meat industry. I wanted to think that my parents were right, because when you're a kid, you want to think your parents make good decisions.

But what were the chances that this was some isolated act of cruelty and abuse? I mean, they call them slaughter-houses for a reason, not euthanasia centers. Even if the depictions of cruelty that I had seen were uncommon, how did I think most of these animals that became bacon and pork chops came to that end? "By being pet to death?" as our friend Vic says. Natural causes? Accidental drug over-dose after a decade of engaging in every kind of depraved excess while touring with their band? *Probably* not.

But, hell, I didn't have to blindly believe my parents. And I didn't have to blindly believe the pamphlet I'd read. I wasn't going to be one of those people who shares an article about how Mr. Rogers wore a necklace of ears from the kills he made in 'Nam as a Navy SEAL using his twenty-four-inch biceps so covered in tattoos that he had to wear ugly zip-up sweaters to conceal them and then be-came a force for nonviolence and children's education and isn't that inspiring and surprising and maybe everyone should know this so let's click "share." I was a dude in the twenty-first century, right? I could Google it if I wanted to. Or I could try Bing, but no one tries Bing. Might as well ask my man Jeeves.

ALEC BALDWIN CAMEO

I typed in the search box "slaughterhouse video." It took me to a PETA video titled *Meet Your Meat*. It's a twelve-minute documentary narrated by Alec Baldwin. It goes through every aspect of the meat industry. It basically takes you behind the closed doors of factory farms and slaughterhouses. Those doors are closed for a reason.

"And what did it reveal?" you ask. Oh, you know, just the most insane, unbelievable shit you can imagine—about the pigs, and a whole lot more about other animals. It showed egg-laying hens confined to tiny cages where they shit all over one another, and cows having their throats slit while fully conscious and screaming as they bleed out.

Wow, I thought to myself. *They really were barbarians hundreds of years ago.*

But then it hit me. *Holy shit! They didn't have cameras back then. This is happening right now!*

Watching the videos had a much bigger impact than seeing the pictures and words in the booklet. I had a bit of a mental breakdown for a few minutes. Tears poured out of my eyes. But it wasn't just the horror of what had happened to those animals that got to me. It was the horror of understanding that I'd been lied to my entire life.

I'd been brought up to think that eating meat made you strong, made you healthy, made you a dutiful son and a pillar of the community. I'd been brought up to think that meat came from enormous ranches like the Ponderosa and that animals either died of old age or were given a painless morphine overdose to send them to the great beyond. But that didn't happen. And that meant that someone had been lying to me for years. People like my parents and the elders in the church and my teachers in school. And if I couldn't trust what they had told me about where meat came from and how the animals were treated to get it, then how the fuck could I trust anything or anyone? Learning about what was real didn't just alter my idea of agribusiness, it altered my idea of who I even was. It turned the world upside down. It made me question everything in life. I realized at that moment that I couldn't trust *anyone*.

And by the end of the video I wanted to die. I was horrified. You could say I was born again. I immediately stopped eating meat. This did not go over incredibly well with my so-traditional-it's-almost-ironic family.

THE ANCIENT, ANCIENT MIDWESTERN RESPONSE TO EATING VEGETARIAN

"Mom, Dad—I can't eat meat anymore," I said, telling them what I'd seen.

"That's crazy," my dad said. If eating meat was so bad, then why did Yeager get a steak with all the trimmings when he broke Mach 1? "The neighbors are going to think you're weird."

"Have you thought this through, dear?" my mom asked. "You know what will happen, don't you, if you stop eating meat? You'll get sick. You'll start losing weight."

"And you don't have much weight to lose," my dad said. "You're maybe 110 pounds, soaking wet. And you're rarely soaking wet. Eat your meat and shower more."

"It's the right thing to do," I said.

So I was just like Chuck Yeager. Though, instead of breaking the sound barrier and shaking out the bugs in top secret military aircraft, I was exploring new ways of eating and experimenting with telling my parents, "No pork chops for me, please." Just thinking about it gives me goose bumps. It's hard to believe that a top historian or writer of narrative nonfiction hasn't been inspired to write a probing and page-turning piece of nonfiction about me.

At the ripe old age of seventeen, I finally decided to man the fuck up and eat my tofu. I ditched supporting all that cruelty done to animals, and moved toward a vegan diet.

FIGHTING AGAINST FUR AND ALSO SOCIAL DECORUM

Did you ever know the smart guy in school? The one who read a lot and was pretty confident that he had all the answers? And if he ever disagreed with someone, he would produce facts and figures and citations and references to obscure books and make everyone look stupid? And what would be the result? He wouldn't convince anyone. Why? Because it was more important to him that everyone else think he was smart than it was for him to persuade anyone. And that was me. I acted like I was the only one with a heart and a conscience in the whole goddamn world. I internalized it all and became, let's just say . . . abrasive. It was almost like it was more important to me to convince everyone I was goddamn woke than it was to change anyone's mind about eating meat.

Once I was at a private banquet dinner for some occasion when a friendly woman wearing a fur coat walked up and sat at our table. While I wasn't an expert enough in fur to know what kind of animal she'd dispatched in order to get that coat, I do remember it was full-length, and what might qualify as a bragging fur coat, a "Look at me! I'm wearing fur" kind of coat. All I could think about was how many animals went insane in their cages or were anally electrocuted to make that coat. A mink coat, for example, would require up to seventy minks be killed to get a complete coat. The same for a sable. If it was a rabbit coat, that would only cost about forty rabbit lives. And if it was chinchilla? That would demand a sacrifice of up to two hundred individual chinchillas. We hadn't even exchanged introductions when I immediately asked in an agitated, accusatory voice, "Is that real fur?"

"Yes," she said, smiling, clearly anticipating that I was asking the question as a prelude to a compliment.

I replied, "You're a murderer!"

Yes, I was a prick back then, too.

"What did you say?" a man, her husband, asked.

"You heard me," I said.

"You need to shut your mouth," he said, motioning for one of the waiters, the largest one, with a cannonball for a head. Mr. Clean's moonlighting gig. "This little punk just called my wife a murderer," he said.

"Did you say that to this lady?" the MBD (massive bald dude) asked.

"Why go to me first? You didn't even ask her if she was a murderer."

"Hey, jerk, do you want me to throw you down the stairs?"

The banquet was on the second floor, and it was only one flight of stairs, but I still didn't want to go down them. He put his hand on my arm to escort me out of the room.

"Fine," I said, shrugging off his hand. "You made your point." I was out the door before they even started serving the salad, prompting my brother, Matt, to no doubt say something smooth like "Well, there goes my ride . . ." before following me out the door.

Did this convince the woman that wearing fur was a bad thing? Probably not. Was this a persuasive argument that illustrated to her the cruelties of the fur industry? Unlikely. Did it teach the people around me some compelling facts about fur as fashion that might prevent them from wearing animal skins or fur as a sartorial choice? Hell no. Even though I'd recently grown a conscience, it seemed more important for me to show everyone that I was a badass crusader than it was for me to actually make much of an impact.

But screaming at strangers isn't nearly as satisfying as screaming at someone you know. So it was a good thing that I had Matt around as a focus for my being an asshole.

BRO VS. BRO

When Matt came home from college for the summer, it was not a good mix. Keep in mind that this was after I'd become an outspoken vegetarian activist, screaming at people at parties and acting surly as shit, and Matt was still a huge meat-eating menace. He was kind of like a comic book villain—the Blob. Under six feet tall, tipping the scales at nearly three hundred pounds, my brother basically sweated Big Mac special sauce. The only reason he wasn't exclusively a carnivore was because he needed to balance out his diet with Cheetos and Funyuns. So just about every interaction we had was like a battle of opposites. Except not quite opposites, because we were both so opinionated and stubborn. That's family for you. One sibling may go to college, but when he comes back, everyone reverts to the time where that same kid stole a toy, and there's going to be hell to pay.

My mom wanted Matt to feel welcome and comfortable at home, for reasons I couldn't possibly fathom as a seventeen-year-old prick, so she made sure to cook dinners that he would like. Here's how that would go:

"Enjoy, beloved family," my mom would say, placing a pot roast with all the trimmings on the table.

"Nothing like a nice plate of torture," I'd say.

"Phil, don't be difficult," my dad said. "Your mom worked hard on this."

"Killing this animal is wrong, but forcing Mom to slow roast her for six hours makes it better?"

"It was more like four hours," my mom said.

"Mom, you're perhaps not focusing on my main point here."

"Phil, you need to just calm down," my dad said. Interesting, because nobody in the history of emotional states ever calmed down when told to do so.

"You're just parroting a bunch of propaganda from PETA," Matt said. "Those people are crazy. They throw blood on people in the streets for wearing fur."

"It's not blood, it's just red paint."

"Okay, so that's not crazy at all, then."

"Phil, why can't you just act like other kids?" my dad asked. "You're being all weird. Other kids eat pot roast."

"And shower," Matt added.

"You know what? Screw this—I'm leaving," I said, walking away from the table.

At the same time, my mom, who was not a complete asshole like I was, also wanted me to feel comfortable and welcome, so she made an effort to prepare some vegan meals for my benefit. Keep in mind that "vegan food" is really a bit of a misnomer. Much of what everyone already eats is vegan: fruits, vegetables, grains, beans, nuts, and seeds. It's not like my mom would serve Matt a huge, steaming bowl of green algae, tree bark, and a ream of printer paper. It was good food.

It was important, however, that my mom not label it as vegan. She could choose something with no meat and no dairy, and it could be totally fucking familiar, but depending on her branding, you'd get vastly different results. For instance:

"Hey, everybody—dinner's ready. Who wants spaghetti with marinara sauce?"

"I do!" Matt would say.

But if we used different language, we'd get different results.

"Hey, everybody—dinner's ready. Who wants vegan noodles?"

"Vegan?!" Matt said, spitting on the floor. "Vegan food is disgusting. I'm not a part of Phil's weird food cult. You can cram that shit with walnuts. I'm going to Taco Bell."

It's the same food!

Could Matt theoretically eat fruit and veggies and seeds? Fuck yeah. But none of that mattered to Matt. He hated the fact that I was a vegan and beyond that he hated all vegans. He especially hated the food, whatever he thought that meant, and would refuse to eat it out of spite. As militant a vegan as I was, Matt was just as rabidly antivegan.

Luckily, my weirdness and belligerence began to fade with age and maturity. I was heavily influenced by the writings of Matt Ball, a well-known animal rights advocate and cofounder of Vegan Outreach. Ball suggested being friendly and engaging, and focusing on "getting people to consider their first step toward compassion, rather than arguing for a specific philosophy or diet." After all, people are more likely to listen when you're not being judgmental or yelling at them.

I know. Not exactly rocket science. But to me, it was a wake-up call. Suddenly, it became important to develop social skills. Maybe I could even use those newfound skills to win some hearts and minds. It was sort of like a pitcher who has a pretty good arm and throws a fastball right by a lot of hitters. Eventually, the hitters start figuring him out. So his coach says, "Maybe try to not throw it as hard as you can, every single time." The pitcher resists, because throwing hard stuff *is what makes him special*! Shit, anyone can throw it slower. How is that good advice? Again, it's a simple thing, this idea that changing the velocity will make it harder for hitters to make contact. But once the pitcher understands this simple thing, the game opens up. And that's when I started mowing hitters down.

SOMETIMES HEROES HAVE FAKE NAMES

It was a Friday afternoon in the spring of 2012. I was doing events in New Orleans, trying to promote awareness about animal cruelty. My intern and I would set up demonstrations involving a giant inflatable puppy burger and then coordinate with the media. I'd just finished my last TV interview and was headed to the airport to get back to my place in West Hollywood when I received a call involving some real superhero action.

"Phil," said Matt Rice, the director of operations for Mercy for Animals, "can we ask you a favor?"

"Shoot," I said.

"We've got an undercover investigator, TJ, who's going to be coming through LA to go over some footage and review a case. Would it be all right if he crashed with you for a day or so?"

"Shit yeah!" I said. I told him where TJ could find a spare key outside my house and that I'd be happy to host him.

Talk about a superstar. Undercover investigators are the heroic motherfuckers who film the videos inside factory farms and slaughterhouses. They literally apply for jobs at these death houses. And when they're hired, they just do the job they're hired to do. But in addition to their regular duties, they go into work each and every day wired with a pinhole-sized hidden camera and small microphone. And they just film what happens, day in and day out.

They film some of the most fucked-up, sadistic abuse your brain can conjure up. But the worst part was the standard practices. Ripping a piglet's testicles out without any pain-killers isn't just something TJ caught on video because he was filming during the one time of the year that some freak accident happened. It's something that happened on a routine basis. People were literally hired to do that for their job.

It's some fucked-up shit, don't you agree?

And due to the nature of the work undercover investigators do, they're unable to tell anyone they come in contact with on a day-to-day basis about who they are and what they do. They have to make up a cover story. So I viewed it as a privilege to be allowed on the inside, to actually meet an undercover investigator during his work. Basically, these people are the most awesome motherfuckers in the world, doing shit I couldn't even imagine in order to make the world a better place.

When I got back from the airport, TJ had already made himself at home on the couch. We talked to each other for a bit, immediately got past the typical small-talk bullshit you go through when you meet someone for the first time, and instantly became best bros.

We headed to a bar, Fat Dog, to grab a few drinks.

I asked him about everything. And it almost seemed therapeutic for him to talk about this shit. Everything he had been doing and seeing had been bottled up inside because he basically had to live two separate lives.

If the workers or owner ever found out who he was and what he was doing, he risked something serious happening to him. Many of the people there were armed. This is some seriously courageous work that not just any random fucker can do. Things got pretty intense before he made his escape.

"I was worried on this one case at a Butterball factory farm," he said.

"Why?"

"They knew something was up. They knew someone was investigating them," TJ said.

"How do you know?"

"Because they told me."

"Why would they tell you?"

"They weren't doing it as a favor. Somehow they knew they had an investigator on the inside. And a few days ago, they called me into the office, and they started asking questions."

"Like what?"

"They said they knew there was an undercover investigator working in the fucking slaughterhouse. They wanted to know if I knew anything."

"No shit? Were you freaked out?"

"Fuck yeah, I was freaked out! I didn't know what was going on. Did they know it was me, and were just trying to sweat a confession? Or were they just asking everybody, hoping someone would spill something? If they were just fishing for information, then my best bet was to shut up. But if they knew it was me, maybe I should say something, like I could cut a deal if they were thinking of beating the shit out of me."

"What did you do?"

"Just acted like I didn't know what the hell they were talking about. Said I'd keep my eyes open for anything weird. But that was enough for me. Had to get the hell out of there."

It was a tough life. Not being able to put down roots. The constant fear that someone might slash your tires or crack you in the back of the head with a baseball bat. But then when he would finish a case and sort of come back to everyday society, he couldn't talk about what he did. Undercover investigators have to make up a story when they meet regular people. Because they never know if the people they're meeting have some sort of connection with animal agriculture interests, or if they just have big mouths.

But the work TJ did was important. And as dedicated as I was to what we were doing, his descriptions of his day-to-day life made me sure it was a job I could never do.

In order to get footage of a factory farm and slaughterhouse, TJ first needed to apply for a job. He normally took any job he could get. And since he was applying for a job at a factory farm or slaughterhouse, basically every job was at least kind of fucked up.

CHICKEN TORTURE (AN INSTRUCTIONAL DESCRIPTION)

He spoke of one job in particular at a chicken slaughterhouse. When the chickens arrived, they were dumped out of their tiny crates and violently hung upside down on shackles by their legs. This process causes many birds to break their legs.

The chickens were then dragged through an electrified water bath. The electrified water didn't render them unconscious. It was just supposed to paralyze them. After that, they were dragged across a blade that cuts their throats while they're still conscious.

And after this, many of the birds would flap around and freak the fuck out. This is where TJ stepped in. At this slaughterhouse he was working as what is called a "backup killer." Yes, that is a job title at slaughterhouses. When he filled out the W-2 form on his taxes, and he had to complete the blank marked "occupation," he had to write in "backup killer." And then probably had to specify that he was not a backup singer for the band The Killers, though that would be an awesome job.

> **WTF:** Backup killers work in horrific conditions and are often paid minimum wage to murder animals all day long.

The backup killer grabs all the chickens that avoided the blade the first time through. He takes his knife and slits the chicken's throat. Then the chicken continues on down the line, where she is dragged through scalding water. Many workers talk about the crazy number of chickens who are still alive when they're dragged through the water. Even after the trauma of having their throat slashed, they are then scalded alive. The chickens who make it this far while still alive are called "red birds" by the meat industry. It happens so much they actually have a name for this shit. And this is what TJ had to endure, day after day after day.

As you can imagine, these are some inspiring mother-fuckers. These are the warriors of our generation. They are in many ways unsung and thankless heroes. Without their courage, meat consumption would not be increasingly viewed as weirder and weirder every year. But due in large part to them, meat consumption is being viewed as weird and weirder. And soon everyone in the world will only al-low it to happen in the corner.

And soon after that everyone will look at the weird person eating meat in the corner and go, "Look at that guy over there. Look what he's eating. What the hell? That's some weird-ass shit. What do we do? I'm scared. I've got kids. I don't want him around them. Should we put him in a home?"

Do we think going undercover inside factory farms and slaughterhouses is something everyone should do? No. Only do it if you are a courageous person who can handle seeing and being a part of some crazy-ass shit.

But do we think everyone should at least watch the

videos these investigators make? Yes. At a minimum, we owe it to the animals, especially if we currently eat or have ever eaten meat, to bear witness to the crazy, fucked-up shit being done to them by our society.

WHEN BACKUP KILLERS RETIRE

About two years later, TJ decided to call it quits. He had spent six years doing undercover work. Matt and I were living in Seattle at the time. We threw a big party on the rooftop of our apartment complex, Collins on Pine, to support him coming back to the regular world. The rooftop had an amazing view of the Seattle skyline and Mount Rainier. We'd just moved to Seattle, and didn't know anyone, but what we did know was that TJ deserved a hell of a send-off. So we put the word out that we were going to be throwing a massive party, charging $10 a head, and that the proceeds would go to benefit local animal advocacy groups. The party sold out in less than twenty-four hours.

TJ's work has led to countless criminal convictions, corporate policy changes, and new laws designed to protect farm animals. He spoke all about his experiences, shared many stories, and inspired everyone. There wasn't a dry eye in the house.

So why did TJ have to do this undercover work? Everyone who looks at the footage that he captured is appalled as fuck. But people like TJ aren't just fighting the battle of bringing information to the public. They're also fighting the information that the slaughterhouses and the corporations are putting out to help promote their message. Or as some people call it, propaganda.

These companies don't go out of their way to show how they confine animals into cages so small they can't turn around. Instead, they show images on their packages of animals roaming around in an open field having the time of their lives. They release PR statements with vague wording like "We don't condone animal abuse," or "We don't promote animal cruelty." If they don't define castrating a pig without painkillers as "abuse" or scalding a chicken alive as "cruelty," then they haven't technically told a lie.

You have companies that are slitting many pigs' throats while they're still fully conscious. But on the other hand, they're releasing statements to the news and to the public where they say they "do not tolerate improper animal treatment." How they word their statement is important. Do they say, "We don't tolerate animals being electrocuted"? No. Do they release a statement saying, "We don't tolerate animals being scalded alive?" No, because then they would have to stop doing that shit. Instead, they say that they don't tolerate "improper animal treatment." But if you think it's *proper* to electrocute chickens and scald them alive, then doing so wouldn't make you guilty of "improper animal treatment." From their perspective, maybe letting chickens walk around on wide-open farm-land would be improper animal treatment, for fuck's sake.

Everyone has their own version of the truth. The big corporations say they're not doing anything cruel, but I suppose that mostly gives you some fucking idea of what they define as "cruelty-free." After learning about this, I decided to start eating vegan. And after starting to eat vegan, I decided to do more to help the animals, more to help my friends, more to help the rest of the world. I started working with people like TJ, people taking an active stand to make the world a better place. I'm no hero, that's for shit sure, but I'm doing what I can for what I think is right. And when you go back to that self-centered prick I used to be, you can see how eating vegan was, on a very small scale, a move in a slightly more heroic direction.

My next move in my vegan evolution was to do combat with my carnivore brother, Matt, and get him to man up and eat some fucking tofu.

Challenge accepted.

CHAPTER 3

MATT'S WAKE-UP CALL: HIS PAST LIFE AS A ZOMBIE

PHIL AND I GREW up as very different people. I'm not surprised that he might use military imagery to describe his experiences, since he was much like a pilot. But one of those maverick pilots that made audacious moves that only worked half the time and who nobody wanted to fly with because he was always calling them murderers. I had a different style. I was more easygoing, more laissez-faire, more likely to use French words in everyday conversation. If he was like a maverick pilot, then I was more like an inflatable raft at a summer lake house. Comfortable, low impact, and maybe a little squishier than it needed to be. But damn—everyone liked that inflatable raft!

THE GREAT GASPY (AND OTHER WAYS TO SAY "MATT WAS FAT")

Growing up, I was never what you'd call *athletic*. I was active, certainly, but I was also husky, a word used more often by parents in place of something like "chubby" or "stout" or "well-marbled." I also had a fairly pronounced case of asthma, which required the use of an inhaler. It was so bad that, when I was about four years old, I had to be taken to the hospital. I just couldn't breathe. It felt like someone (probably Phil) was sitting on my chest. The doctors just chalked it up to the fact that Tennessee, where we were living at the time, had a lot of allergens. They gave me my first inhaler and told me to only use it in case of emergencies. I would use that "emergency" inhaler pretty much every day of my life.

By my first year of college, I was tipping the scales at five ten, 265 pounds. I didn't wear it well. I was awkward, lonely, and unhappy. I was still living at home, commuting to school every day. When you're a freshman and you're still living at home, you never feel fully included. You're not bonding with people in a residence hall or a fraternity. It's like you're just a temp. Don't get too attached to that guy—he'll be heading home soon. And make sure he doesn't steal any staples or Post-it notes.

At the same time, a stranger looking at me from the outside wouldn't have a clue that I was having a tough time, because I put a shitload of energy into being loud and extroverted and funny. Because if you're the one making people laugh, then you're making a contribution. And if you're contributing, there's less incentive for someone to say, "Why are you so gross and fat?" I was like the social version of Rudy. I needed to show these people that I belonged, and I was going to accomplish that through sheer force of will. I wanted to lose weight, but when you grow up believing that at least two meals per day have to contain a significant amount of meat in order to count as "nutritious," then you're kind of behind the eight ball. And also I resembled an eight ball.

SCHOOL DAZED AND FAT AS FUCK

My days at Eastern Michigan University revolved around food—a lot of food. The menu for breakfast was an obscene amount of McDonald's. (Yes, both Vegan Bros were addicted to that Mickey D's smack.) After a class or two, I'd hit up the Taco Bell in the EMU food court (we literally had fast food inside the campus!) for six tacos, two orders of churros, and a Dr Pepper the size of a newborn. Next up would be an afternoon "snack" at the Great Steak and Potato Company, where I would annihilate three thousand calories in a few minutes. Dinner consisted of two entire frozen pizzas and an ice-cream-laden, whole-milk chocolate shake. And then for a late-night snack I'd hit up Taco Bell again. In fact, I like to think I helped inspire Taco Bell's late-night-snack menu, known officially as "Fourth Meal." The problem with this claim, though, is that this was actually my fifth meal of the day. Gross.

I'd estimate that back then I consumed upward of seven thousand calories per day. I suffered from hypertension and depression. I was alive, but not living. I was a zombie, except zombies have more friends. And probably eat a slightly healthier diet. At least most of the items on the zombies' menu are free-range.

At this point, I knew something had to give. All my friends from the church my brother and I grew up in had moved away. I felt I wasn't really starting the next phase of my life or moving forward so much as treading water, and I decided to transfer, ending up at Evangel University, or EU, as no one calls it. Evangel, in lovely Springfield, Missouri—the buckle of the Bible belt—is just one step below a full-fledged Bible college. I had to take required church classes and attend mandatory Sunday church and chapel at school three hours per week. No drinking or sex was allowed, which was a major buzzkill. Being a nearly three-hundred-pound sophomore transfer who had permanent chalupa breath, I was accustomed to bumping uglies with the coeds. Often, I'd be plagued by three, sometimes four gorgeous communications majors saying, "Please, Matt! Take us to bed or lose us forever!" And I'd say, "Sorry, ladies, but if there is one thing I believe in, it's EU's conduct code. And if there's another thing I believe in, it's the sleepwalker's menu at Denny's, so I must be on my way."

Even on a new campus, I felt like my life was tied down by an anchor. As the old saying goes: wherever you go, there you are. I woke up each morning feeling lethargic and sick. I was going through the motions: go to class, eat, do homework, eat, take exams, eat. I had no expectations for life. No ambitions. No goals. I had begun keeping a journal. That's when you know shit is really bad.

And even worse, I wasn't the only person who thought I was gross and pathetic. My dad had also somehow figured out this secret. He was a somewhat intense guy, and it bothered him that I was overweight and undertall. He didn't mince words.

"Matt, you like going to EU?"

"Yeah, it's fine."

"It's costing me a pretty penny."

"I know. And thanks, by the way, for paying the tuition. Really appreciate it."

"You know I'm not paying that tuition just so you can keep Domino's and the Cheesecake Factory in business, right? So if you don't change things, then I might have to."

"Wait—what?"

"I'm paying for you to get an education. Not diabetes."

"Yeah, well, that's a little harsh, but . . ."

"Lose some weight or pay your own tuition."

"But, Dad—what if I'm just naturally a heavy guy?"

45

"Then I guess you're going to have to find a job that doesn't require a lot of wind sprints."

Click.

So I resolved to make a change.

Mostly by lying to my dad. All great revolutions begin with lying to your parents. Thomas Jefferson once skipped a cousin's wedding so he could write a draft of the Declaration of Independence, but told his family that he really just had a severe attack of gout (which, incidentally, is a condition caused by the consumption of organ meats and so rarely affects vegans). Prior to the Bolshevik Revolution, Lenin stole his father's hammer and sickle to loan to an aspiring flag designer, saying, "I think some kids swiped them as part of a high school prank." And Han Solo, before blasting Darth Vader off that trench of the Death Star, visited his parents (the Solos, which is funny) and told them that he needed a few bucks to help pay off Jabba the Hutt, when really he had plenty of reward money and blew his parents' cash on vests.

So every few weeks, I would tell my dad, "Hey, Pop, I lost another five pounds. Doing lots of ultimate Frisbee," and "Looking forward to seeing you guys at Thanksgiving. I'll show off my new belt—the only way to keep these super-baggy pants up!" But it's not like I could keep that going forever. I wasn't going to school in Indonesia, for fuck's sake.

At my lowest point, I asked God for help. I begged for a way to turn around my pathetic, dead-end life.

My first step on that road? Sitting on my palatial ass and watching a movie.

Hey, from tiny acorns do mighty oaks grow, right?

That movie was *Super Size Me*, the Morgan Spurlock documentary about his personal experiences with the fast-food industry. Spurlock decided to eat exclusively at McDonald's for a month to see how it would affect his body, his mood, and his life. It did not go well.

After thirty days, Spurlock had gained almost twenty-five pounds and saw his cholesterol skyrocket, his libido plunge, and depression begin to set in. His doctor observed that Spurlock appeared to have an addiction to fast food, and though consuming it would give him a brief high, it would also plunge him into feelings of withdrawal. Spurlock also exhibited the beginning of liver disease, and so ended his experiment after thirty days, convinced that eating a lot of fast food wouldn't just be a poor diet for someone training for the Olympics, but that it would actually kill him.

That was some eye-opening shit.

I mean, I was eating a diet that wasn't dramatically different than the one that Spurlock put himself on. And in a month, it almost killed the guy. Maybe this was a sign that I should take a closer look at my fast-food intake.

Did I want to be depressed? To have no libido? To die of high cholesterol and some combination of heart and liver disease?

Hell no!

TAKING A STAND

So I gave it up. No more Taco Bell. No more Domino's. No more McDonald's or Wendy's or Burger King or KFC. Would that change things for me? At my lowest point, I'd just sit in my room, ordering Papa John's (the most depressing of the cheap delivery pizzas) and scarf down an entire pie with some cheese sticks and a huge soda. Those days were now over. If I gave it up, then I might lose fifty pounds. Maybe eighty, if things really went my way.

It didn't quite work out like I'd hoped.

I lost about seven pounds.

That might not seem like much. Just seven measly pounds. But sometimes, a little can be a lot. Losing seven pounds proved that I could lose the weight if I made a change. It proved that I wasn't trapped for the rest of my life. And all that I'd given up was fast food.

That moment opened the floodgates for me. But I still had a ways to go. After all, I had not yet fully committed to vegan eating. I was still morbidly obese. I still felt conspicuous when hanging out with friends as the fat impostor that needed to prove his worth. And I was going to a

Bible college when I wasn't necessarily ready for a career in the Bible industry.

What I'd done had been a pretty simple, pretty minor change. What if I did more? What if I made more of an effort to eat a healthy diet? And work out? Could I expect even more dramatic gains, and losses, if I did that? There was one problem.

I didn't know shit about diet or working out or losing weight.

But I knew someone who did.

WHEN A FATTY NAMED MATTY ASKS FOR HELP

With a little wind in my sails, I got up the courage to ask the most ripped guy I knew if he could help me at the gym. Andy Zart played on the defensive line for the EU football team (the Crusaders, in case the student body didn't realize it was a Christian university) and was a pretty jacked six four and 240. He lived in the same residence hall that I did, just six doors down.

Keep in mind, it wasn't easy to ask Andy to help me exercise. When I was younger, the idea of being the fat kid changing in the locker room and getting made fun of or taking a lot of shit in gym class made me get a note from my doctor that got me out of gym. The gym is not tradi- tionally my place of refuge. But desperate times called for desperate measures.

"Hey, Andy, you're pretty in shape, right?"

"I'm a brick shithouse. I eat lightning and crap thunder."

"Great. So could you give me some help? Maybe some pointers on how to get a good sweat going?"

He extended his hand toward me and placed a single pebble from the floor onto his palm. "First, take the pebble from my hand. Then I'll know you are ready."

"What?"

"Nah. I'm just messing with you. The trick to exercise is going to the gym."

It was true—he *did* know secrets I could barely fathom!

But, hey, it's what I needed. I was desperate, and he was willing to help a brother out.

That help included workout tips, an individualized regimen, and literally getting directions on where to find the gym since I had never set foot in one. Once we got there, Andy started taking me through a pretty standard workout of free weights, hitting the bench press and inclined press, doing curls, squats, and flys. It was going pretty well, and I was getting a good sweat going, when I felt something. It seemed that the revolution I had begun with my muscles was meeting heavy resistance from the bologna-and-mayo sandwich I'd eaten for lunch. I put the curl bar I'd been lifting on the floor and told Andy, "Just a second, bro," and ran to a door leading outside the fitness center. I'd just gotten outside when I hurled all over the ground.

It was winter, so steam was everywhere. It was coming from my breathing, coming off my sweat-soaked T-shirt, coming off the puke I'd yakked on campus. It was like everything about me was on fire. Maybe it was too much. Maybe this was a sign I should stop. But maybe it was a sign that there were parts of me that *needed* burning down. And, shit, I didn't want Andy to think I was a little bitch.

I thought about how I felt then, thought about how I usually felt, and went back in.

"Glad to have you back," Andy said.

"Sorry about that," I replied.

"No worries, Matt. Pain is just the feeling of weakness leaving the body."

"Weakness and some bologna," I corrected. Puking was gross, but it was kind of fascinating to watch food actually go *out* of my mouth for once.

> **FUN FACT:** Strength training changes the way your body works. For every pound of muscle tissue added, your body burns an average of an extra fifty calories per day just because it's there. AKA burning fat while you veg out on the couch.

Andy admired my moxie and went to the gym with me every day for two weeks. He didn't teach me anything crazy or technical, just a lot of weight lifting and a lot of treadmill, stationary bike, and elliptical machine. But I stuck with it. On day fifteen, the training wheels came off, and I was on my own.

Once I got rolling, it was hard to stop me (last fat joke). I became a gym rat. And with encouragement and guidance from Phil, instead of head-bashing rhetoric, my diet vastly improved as well. I was still eating meat, but I was definitely eating healthier than I had been previously. Day by day. One foot in front of the other.

HE LOST IT ALL . . .

After one year of working out and eating right, I had lost a hundred pounds. This is an important detail. Yeah, I lost a shitload of weight, but I didn't lose it in a day or a week or a month. It took a year of dedicated effort to lose a hundred pounds. Lots of times, people will want to lose weight or become a vegan and get fucking depressed when it doesn't happen in the same week that they made their decision. That's the hard part. Some of these things take time. And people need to embrace that time. They don't have to feel like they're behind if they don't get dramatic effects in a narrow time period. Don't be in a rush. It's a process and you just have to embrace the process.

You know what happens when you try to rush things? You get yo-yo diets, and nothing really changes long-term.

When I came home after graduating college, people

didn't even recognize me. People would literally stare at me, like they were wondering, "Is that guy a celebrity? Or a fugitive from *America's Most Wanted*? Why do I know that face?" Lots of double takes from people I had known for fucking *years*. I had begun to question all of the religious and political paradigms foisted upon me by the church and, even worse, the meat industrial complex. It was incredibly empowering. I realized I could do anything. I'd lost a hundred pounds. I'd shed a couple of chins. I now had a jawline. My body had transformed itself, like a superhero or a sort of reverse puffer fish. I felt like I had actually lived as two different people, transforming into my more powerful, dynamic self after hitting the gym. The change was good.

Maybe I could even change something that was dramatically affecting my life.

Specifically, breathing.

But I'd need Phil's help.

BREAKTHROUGH

One day, Phil had casually, politely, and subtly mentioned a documentary he was interested in, and I decided to flip it on. Keep in mind, Phil did not do polite or subtle. If Phil were to play poker, he would say shit like, "I raise you one hundred dollars, and I'm also bluffing like a motherfucker." This was a bit of a problem when we were growing up. Phil would find something he cared about, and because he was a passionate dude, he'd try to convince other people that they should get on board. But because we're both strong-willed people, I had an almost reflexive sense of "If I do what he says, then it means I'm weaker than he is, and I lose and he wins, and I'm not going to do that." So we'd have these kinds of conversations:

"Hey, Matt, you should be a vegan."

"Oh, really? Fuck off."

"Seriously, dude. It's the right way to be."

"Damn, Phil, stop pushing so hard! I feel like I'm the only guy in a bus station at two a.m. and you're trying to sell me Amway shit."

"You need to stop being so passive and stand up to the meat industry!"

"I am standing up to someone. You. Go eat a spotted owl and stop bothering me."

He would push something at me, and I'd just push back twice as hard. So it was when Phil said something that didn't involve me having to wrestle with him that I finally got a little perspective. Phil mentioned that there was a documentary that he really wanted to see, but that it was on HBO and he didn't have HBO. He wasn't ramming it down my throat. Maybe that was it. Maybe it was that he wasn't giving me the hard sell. Maybe it was that he wanted to watch this thing, and because he couldn't, it made it more appealing to me. I could see something that he couldn't. So I decided to check it out.

It was March 2009 and the documentary was *Death on a Factory Farm*.

In the film, an undercover investigator secretly records severe and illegal abuse at a pig farm in Ohio. I was caught off guard and watched with an open mind for perhaps the very first time. I watched as they hung pigs upside down by a forklift until they choked to death and whipped a pig with broken legs to make her move. In that moment, I connected not with the one doing the whipping, but with the ones being whipped.

I broke down in sobs. It was almost a relief to finally let those fucking tears flow. They were tears of sadness not just for my own situation, but for the billions of animals with no voice or choice who die each year just to get on our plates. It felt like the wool had been pulled over my eyes all these years. As Paul McCartney famously said, "If slaughterhouses had glass walls, we'd all be vegetarian." And Sir Paul McCartney is always right, because he's a Beatle, and, well, that's really all we need to say about that.

And it's not just pigs. Do you know what happens to cows? Most cows are born on dairy farms and ripped from their mother immediately after birth. They're born one day, and stolen the next.

Momma cows love their little babies. And they freak out when their babies are taken. They cry for weeks. It's depressing as hell to hear the cries.

But the worst part is where the babies are sent. They're

transported to veal farms, where they're chained by the neck inside crates barely larger than their own bodies, living in their own feces. Talk about luxury.

They're slaughtered when they're just sixteen weeks old. Talk about some weird, fucked-up shit.

There's a reason that they call baby cows "veal": because putting "baby cow" on a menu in a four-star restaurant would probably have an adverse effect on the evening's receipts.

It doesn't sound real, does it? Well, it is.

And having her baby calf stolen from her isn't the only bad thing that happens to the momma cow. Cows produce milk for their babies. But the baby was sent to a veal farm, so the farmers end up taking that shit.

And they want to keep that milk production going. So they do this to her over and over. They artificially and repeatedly inseminate the cows. And dairy cows are barely given any room to move, either. After around three years, they're sent to slaughter.

Cows aren't the only animals forced to endure these kinds of cruel and inhumane treatments. Fish suffer, too.

"Fish?" you say. "Who cares about fish? Baby cows have big eyes and shy smiles and are innocent and adorable and fish are alien and weird and kind of beneath my contempt." And it's true that fish *are* kind of weird looking, which makes them harder to empathize with. But that doesn't mean that they don't deserve some compassion, right?

The experts agree that fish are intelligent and feel pain.

And they also experience pleasure. So the shit we do to them matters.

And you may be thinking, *But I just cast my rod out, hook the fish in the face, he or she writhes in pain trying to get away, I pull the fish from the water with the hook still in the face, then I take the fish, skin him or her alive, and then I eat him or her.*

That's kind of fucked up. But it's nowhere near as fucked up as what they do to fish sold in most restaurants and grocery stores.

One of the ways they do it is with mile-long nets. They take those things and drag them along the ocean floor. And they catch anything and everything, including dolphins and turtles. And then when they bring the nets up, there's a change in pressure. So the fish undergo excruciating decompression, which divers know as "the bends," where many of them have their swim bladders ruptured, while others have their eyes pop out.

They're then dumped onto the ship, where they're either crushed to death or suffocated. And still some are alive while they're hacked to death.

One in five fish consumed in the world come from captivity. These places are known by many as "aquatic factory farms." These fish are confined by the tens of thousands in tiny areas filled with feces for their entire lives. They're eventually loaded up on a massive truck and shipped to slaughter. Common killing methods include slow suffocation.

It's a really good time.

So I bid adios to meat.

Really, it was just the next logical step. I'd given up fast food, and lost some weight. I started working out and eating more fruits and veggies, and lost a ton more weight. So on the continuum of being healthy, putting an end to my meat eating was just the next stop on my journey. Well, that and saying shit like "It was the next stop on my journey." Those things go hand in hand.

Not long after I'd given up eating meat, our mom did as well, then our dad. This was huge, since our dad equated eating meat with inhaling oxygen. If you didn't take it in, you couldn't be healthy. Maybe because of his becoming a vegetarian, our extended family did, too (except our fish-clubbing grandfather, but no one is perfect).

I was feeling a lot better. I was working out every day, I looked and felt a lot better than I used to, but there was one problem.

I still had trouble breathing.

WAITING TO INHALE

I grew up with severe allergies and asthma. I had to puff a rescue inhaler three to four times per day and was using a steroid twice daily. It was no fun.

Even after I started eating better, the symptoms persisted. I'd lost a lot of weight, so I had hoped that I'd get my breathing under control. After all, I was hauling around a lot less bulk, and I was more fit than I'd ever been in my life. How come I couldn't breathe? I would always need another puff or two from my "emergency" inhaler, and it was only ten a.m. This inhaler, which I was told to use only for emergencies, I would have to use every couple of hours every single day just to breathe normally.

I was getting sick and tired of taking all of these prescription drugs to counteract my symptoms.

"I want to get to the root of the problem," I told my doctor. I was a big fan of Dr. George. I'd met him at the Michigan veg fest, and he seemed to know his shit.

Dr. George said, "Try cutting out dairy and see what happens. You might be surprised."

The underlying argument he made was that I might have a food allergy, specifically an allergy to dairy. When most people think of food allergies, they imagine something like the dramatic reaction that some people have to peanuts, where eating a single peanut can send someone (like me, for example, who is also fucking deathly allergic to peanuts) into anaphylactic shock. The consumption produces an immediate reaction that helps to identify the allergy. But not all food allergies are the same. Some allergies can take hours, or even days, to produce an effect. As a result, the person suffering from the allergy won't attribute the allergy attack to something they ate days before. Instead, they'll think, *Shit, I can't breathe. Better take a hit from my inhaler.* And one of the foods that might produce this kind of reaction: dairy.

According to Physicians Committee for Responsible Medicine (PCRM), at least 75 percent of the world's population alone is intolerant to some form of dairy, where their bodies don't produce enough of an enzyme (lactase) necessary for breaking down lactose, the sugar found in most dairy products. This can cause gas pains (farts, to those not fluent in euphemism), bloating, cramps, and diarrhea (the shits, amigo). And many others are actually allergic, where their bodies have a specific allergic reaction to dairy.

I couldn't get what Dr. George said out of my head. I'd already cut out butter, dairy milk, and whey protein, so all I had left to go was cheese.

And so I did it. I cut out cheese. Which at first was no easy task. I love cheese. Pizza, nachos, mozzarella sticks, grilled cheese—these are a few of my favorite things. I didn't want to give them up. But there was something that was arguably even more important that I also didn't want to give up: air. So I put an embargo on the cheese.

Before going off cheese, I'd routinely use the rescue inhaler three to six times *per day* just to keep up.

Get this.

Within three days I wasn't using this inhaler *at all*.

My inhaler was now serving the purpose for which it was designed: emergencies. I only required its use a couple of times per year. My life had completely been transformed.

I used to walk around with an indentation in my left side pocket from carrying that inhaler around, like it was my lifeline. Now I would go months without using it. After I started breathing so much better, I ditched the steroid that I'd been taking as well. I'd been ingesting that shit for five years, and as soon as I went off dairy, I just left it in the medicine cabinet. Good riddance.

It was amazing. All my life, I'd been seeing allergists, asthma specialists, and doctors of all types in an effort to get a hold of my asthma problem. Not *one* of them had ever suggested that I might need to alter my fucking diet. Why hadn't that come up? I'd had asthma my whole life, but it wasn't like I was carting a Persian cat with me everywhere I'd go, to college, to work, to the toilet. I didn't have a thirty-year exposure to bee pollen. Why was it that they kept asking the same questions? Why had no one ever asked about what kind of food I ate? I don't want to get all conspiracy theory, but it makes you wonder about the influence of the meat-dairy industrial complex. And also chemtrails, and the flat earth theory.

Now, this isn't to say if you have asthma or allergies that dairy is the main cause. But it very well could be.

Of course, everyone's experience will be different and we don't promise miracles. You will not turn into a ten and start scoring supermodels overnight (it could take a few weeks). Many vegans report that their skin clears up and appears more vibrant and younger-looking. This is known as the fabled "vegan glow." Some studies show that vegans taste better (it's an oral thing). That's right: lovers have reported that their vegan partners actually taste better than omnivorous ones. That alone may be a reason to give this a try.

When people start eating more vegetables than they used to, they end up getting more essential minerals and nutrients. That can lead to better sleep, more energy, and even, well, better sex. It's true: vegans do it better.

Now that my health was more in order, I began asking myself that eternal question: What the fuck am I going to do with my life? I had no plan for when college ended. I was just passively thinking that I'd get a degree, and then a job would just sort of materialize. But what job did I even want to get?

FROM CHURRO TO GURU

A mentor of mine, a family friend named Dennis Whaley (who was also the head of PR for my college), noted my recent physical transformation and suggested I take a look at the fitness industry. "Hey," he said to me half jokingly, "you could be the next Richard Simmons."

This suggestion was actually not far from something I'd already considered. I knew I wanted to help people transform their lives just like I had. So I wrote a business plan, took out a small business loan, and opened my first gym right near our hometown in Howell, Michigan. The guy who in high school would get doctor's notes to get out of gym now owned one.

I learned that I found it more stimulating to start a business than run one. So I sold the gym and started another. Then I heard about a gym that was going south, so I sold the one I owned and bought that third gym, and in a month managed to make it turn a profit. The business was flourishing, but still I wished there was something even more directly I could do to help people improve themselves. I became a personal trainer, enabling me to have an even closer relationship with my clients and to counsel them not just on exercise and weight loss, but also nutrition, diet, and lifestyle. Many of them even became vegans as well. Still, I felt unfulfilled. There were only so many people I could reach from a small town in Michigan. I wanted to have a bigger, more global impact, but I had no idea how.

I'd lost a hundred pounds, become vegan, gotten a ripped physique, cleared up a debilitating asthma condition, become a fitness mogul, and discovered a sense of purpose to do something more important for the world. And now I wanted to help the world. I may not have been a hero, but my heart was in the right place. Now I just needed a cause.

I'd find it in a four-month-old named Peyton.

CHAPTER 4

MR. PEYTERSON:
A BOY AND HIS DOG

Life was good for Matt. Money was coming in at a good clip and he was feeling like he was actually helping the world a bit, contributing to people getting healthier, sharing his wisdom about diet and exercise with his clients. He had launched his first gym to fanfare and almost instantaneous success in 2008. Incredibly, the success came in the face of the worst economic downturn in years, in one of the hardest-hit states in the country, Michigan. Sometimes, the most tenacious plants take root in even the most inhospitable soil.

Matt's other upside was scoring a sick bachelor pad for half price. That didn't benefit humanity as much, unless you factor in the benefit it gave to liquor retailers (and on a good night, wholesalers) and party supply stores. The amount of money he spent on tap insurance alone was staggering.

It was a 2,600-square-foot, three-story, completely upgraded townhouse with hardwood floors, appliances by manufacturers he'd never even heard of, and plenty of room for activities (*Step Brothers*, anyone?).

He invited two of his best friends, Eric and Danny, to become his roommates, and it quickly became the most banging postcollege frat house ever. It had all the trappings, including a Ping-Pong table in the kitchen, tastefully upgraded with tile.

Almost every weekend there'd be pre-parties with beer pong tournaments and a keg on the deck, often emptied before midnight. Keg stands, flip cup, full rock band set up in the living room, and always fifteen to fifty of our closest friends.

With theme parties like '80s night, CEOs and Randos, and the always epically executed Halloween parties (equipped with a fully functional smoke machine), we had a blast.

We've all been to those parties where it's BYOB, or pay to drink. We didn't believe in that shit. We took care of our damn guests, and that meant food, drinks, everything.

DRINK AND BE VEGAN

If the thing you prioritize in your partying is finding a loud carnivore and bro-ing down on your shared interest in drinking excessively and enjoying your weekend, there's good news: there are plenty of loud vegans who love the same shit.

It was a fact that we liked to party. And we did our parties right.

The point is if you're as sick of hearing from all of the self-righteous "nothing bad goes in my body and it shouldn't go in yours either" shit, then you're in the right place.

Are we saying alcohol is healthy?

Hell no.

Are we saying Oreos are healthy, for that matter? NO.

But they're both vegan. Got it?

> **FUN FACT:** Double Stuf Oreos are delicious. AND vegan.

So if you like kicking ladies' night with your girlfriends watching *The Bachelor* and sipping on some wine: that shit's stone-cold vegan.

If you're in a frat and you rage seven days a week instead of going to class and being responsible, guess what? That's vegan as fuck.

If you like hitting up trendy and hip cocktail bars and speakeasies for an old-fashioned: vegan.

Or maybe you're on a tropical vacation and you want a mai tai. Drink that vegan deliciousness up.

If you love vodka on the rocks with a lime (like us), then you belong on a Go Vegan poster, because that shit is vegan.

Basically, you can party as hard as you want. Connect with your friends. Rage at the frat. Tear it up at the family reunion. Toast the bride and groom over and over and over again. Be the flip cup, quarters, or beer pong champion. It's all good. And it's all vegan.

Unless you're a weirdo having a bacon martini (and we're sure someone's drinking one right now), most alcohol is vegan. Avoid the White Russians and drinks with milk in them, or simply replace the 2 percent milk with some coconut milk, and you'll be toasted *and* vegan.

Being vegan doesn't mean you can't have fun. It doesn't mean you have to always make healthy decisions or that you won't wake up on a Sunday morning and regret things you did on Saturday night. Vegans love to party, and eating vegan doesn't mean you have to give up vodka, beer, or Sour Patch Kids. Live it up!

Phil was in college about forty-five minutes away at Michigan State, but would visit on weekends and sufficiently tore shit up each time he was there, often passing out on an inflatable bed in the home office, or on the floor in the kitchen underneath all the couch cushions we stacked on top of him.

It was good times.

And it's not like the parties stopped once the weekend was over. Nothing going on Tuesday? Sounds good. Let's have ten people over for a midweek vodka-fueled excuse to get drunk. You bored on a Thursday? Come on over for a drunk round-robin Ping-Pong tourney.

As fun as all of this was, Matt started to feel like there was something missing. He had money. He had friends. He was dating a ton. But he felt a certain emptiness, a certain loneliness. He wasn't ready to settle down and have kids, but he was ready for another kind of commitment—he wanted a dog.

HOME IS WHERE THE BARK IS

Growing up with our family pets Lillie (miniature poodle) and Skyler (cairn terrier) always seemed to be the finishing touch in making a house feel like home. And they weren't at Matt's bachelor mansion. Lillie was our first family dog. She had black curly hair and a thin tail with a big black puff at the end like a 1980s microphone. She was an energetic, happy ball of joy.

Lillie was part of the house before either of us arrived on the scene. For a couple of years, it was just her and our parents. Matt came next. It must have been a trip for her—having free rein over the house, and then suddenly there's this little annoying, noisy, chubby kid crawling around, screaming and poking her. Lillie must have had the patience of a saint. Then, for the few years before Phil was born, she was Matt's only friend. She wasn't just a dog—she was a part of the family.

We'd head to one side of the house with Lillie jumping around demanding we throw her a ball. Then we'd throw it over the roof, all the way to the other side. She knew exactly what to do.

We always wanted to bring her with us wherever we went. We'd get upset and protest when we were going to the store and she couldn't come. We still feel like that to this day. We maintain that dogs should be able to go everywhere people can. And why can't they? Because they might leave dog hair? Fun science fact: Phil has more germs in one knee pit than most dogs have on their entire bodies. Phil is disgusting. And he's allowed in most restaurants and shops!

Lillie eventually got old and was diagnosed with pancreatic cancer. One day we came home from school and she could barely move. Her health had been deteriorating for the last few months. But this was by far the worst we'd seen her.

The vet had directed us to have corn syrup on hand to help spike her blood sugar when she was low. She'd lick it from the spoon as we'd pet her and tell her, "It's going to be okay."

Usually, within twenty minutes or so, she'd begin to perk up. But this time nothing happened. The corn syrup didn't seem to have any positive effect on her. We waited a bit to see if she would improve. But this time was different. We eventually drove her to the vet.

We hoped and almost assumed the best. She was going to get well enough to be able to come home. But when we woke up the next morning, she was gone. "She died, peacefully, in her sleep," the veterinarian said.

It was the first close experience with death for both of us. And it was hard. She wasn't just a dog—she was a part of the family. We took trips together. We played ball. We went for walks. She would lie with us when we were sick.

She was our first introduction to the love, companionship, and empathy a human can feel for an animal.

The bond between her and Matt would lead to a more profound awe and appreciation for animals.

After Lillie's passing there was a big void in the Letten household. A void all four of us felt. So we began the search. At the time, the only way we considered finding our next best friend was from a breeder, though we learned a lot during the search and ended up being exposed to the dark puppy mill industry (more on that shortly).

Eventually we welcomed Skyler into our home. Matt was in eighth grade, Phil in fifth. Skyler was the smartest dog we had ever met. He grew up with us. We taught him sit, shake, roll over, crawl, dance—you name it, he could do it. He even learned to yawn on command. He loved running and exploring in the woods, occasionally leaving us frantically running around calling for him, as he had a habit of chasing after squirrels.

When we both left for college, Skyler stayed back and hung with our parents. We'd return often and pick up right back where we left off. He lived a long healthy life, but around sixteen he started losing weight. By seventeen he was very sick. We felt terrible. Our best friend was struggling. Our mom did her best to keep Skyler happy and comfortable, but shortly after we rang in the 2016 New Year he took a nose dive. Matt happened to be in town, and with our dad and mom made the difficult but necessary decision to go to the animal hospital.

They bawled their eyes out, loving on Skyler one last time, and were there to see him off as the medicine took over. It never gets easier to lose family.

Fast-forward just over ten years and Matt was walking a new path. He'd given up meat, had gone vegan, and was more aware than ever about how important animal lives were. While those lives were at greatest risk from the companies that converted animals into food, there was another group that threatened animals with torture and death—people who converted pets into profit.

BRED FOR CASH

According to the Humane Society of the United States (HSUS), as of May 2016 there were an estimated ten thousand puppy mills. This included both licensed and unlicensed breeders. The ASPCA defines a puppy mill as "a large-scale commercial dog breeding operation where profit is given priority over the well-being of the dogs." These places don't view dogs as living, thinking creatures, but as product. Their goal isn't to match a puppy with the right companion, but to sell an animal for the most money while spending the bare minimum on his needs. All the incentives for these piece-of-shit commercial kennel operators are to deprive the dogs of their physical and emotional needs.

The HSUS estimates that over ninety-nine thousand female dogs are used solely for the purpose of breeding as many dogs as they can. They have miserable lives trapped in cages, moving from pregnancy to pregnancy and then repeatedly having their puppies torn from them. The ASPCA recommends that mothers remain with their litters for eight to ten weeks, but for dogs produced at these mills and kennels, puppies can be taken away with almost no time shared between parent and offspring.

HSUS has reported that around two and a half *million* healthy dogs and cats are euthanized in shelters each year. Over two million. Can you really imagine the magnitude of that number of lives lost? That's more than the number of stone blocks in the Great Pyramid at Giza. That's more than the number of pounds in a redwood tree. It's over ten times the distance, in miles, to the moon. The euthanizing of these animals is due to pet overpopulation, perpetuated by greedy breeders interested in padding their pockets while they mistreat and abuse their animals. These breeders aren't matchmakers—they don't find the perfect dog for the perfect family. The perfect dog is any dog they can sell, and the perfect family is a family that will pay cash.

And their puppies? Due to overbreeding, unhealthy conditions, and often inbreeding, puppy mill animals have been shown to have more health problems than an average dog. Hip dysplasia, pneumonia, mange, giardia, and heartworm are all common afflictions for these dogs. Do you know what mange is? It sounds like it's a bad haircut, but it's a skin disease caused by parasitic mites devouring helpless dogs. And you might think that heartworms are just microscopic little bugs that don't seem all that scary, but they're actually foot-long worms that can live in a dog's heart and lungs. How many foot-long worms can live in a dog's vital organs? If untreated, a dog can have literally *hundreds* feeding off its body. That shit is fucked up.

Dogs are often trapped twenty-four hours a day in crowded cages stacked on top of one another. They're forced to shit and pee all over the place. They're rarely fed properly, and never get routine humane veterinary checkups.

Because they're raised basically in a canine version of *The Matrix*, born in a cage and living in their own piss and shit, dogs are both unhealthy and often poorly socialized. They suffer from pains both physical and psychological. And if you think dogs can't have psychological problems, you've never seen a puppy crying and whimpering at the sight of a goddamn brown loafer because someone used to throw shoes at him every time he made a noise.

> **FUN FACT:** Over a third of families in the United States own a dog.

Breeders may start out with the best of intentions, but when profits get in the way, those intentions often slip away entirely.

These breeders are running an assembly line. The more products you push through, the more you get paid. They don't care about the lives of each dog they're neglecting and torturing on a daily basis. Just the almighty dollar. (For the record, we think money is awesome. But making money from animal abuse is not okay.)

FRANKENPUPS

Even more disturbing, on some levels, is what happens to animals at the higher levels of the for-profit pet industry, with "legitimate" breeders determined to produce dogs showcasing the apex of what their breed should be. This can create inbred and unhealthy animals. For instance, dachshunds are prized for their length, and wiener dogs are sure as shit adorable, but when taken to the extreme, this produces dogs that have unnaturally long backs that create back and hip problems that can be agonizing for the dog. Bulldogs are bred to have flat faces, and so breeders have emphasized this trait to such an extreme that the resulting bulldogs can find breathing almost impossible. The skulls of some of these animals are so huge, their mothers can't give birth to them without surgical intervention. The creation of these Frankendogs is both unnatural and cruel.

TAKING A STAND FOR PUPS

After learning about some of these practices while doing research about the moral and ethical conundrums of raising animals for livestock, Matt made a realization. "I have to do something," he thought. "This shit is fucked up." And let's face it, that dude was dog sick. He needed some puppy love in his life.

He filled out an application to foster with a nationwide dog rescue group, Cairn Rescue USA (CRUSA). First we had to complete an interview and background check. Their representative arrived to inspect Matt's living conditions and make sure he wasn't some nutcase.

"Have you always loved animals?" the woman, Rhonda, asked.

"Absolutely. I grew up with dogs, and I'm a huge animal lover. Hell, part of the reason that everyone here doesn't eat meat is because we love animals. Just not with a side of fries, if you know what I mean," Matt said.

"Wait, who doesn't eat meat?"

"Me," Matt said. "And my brother Phil there." Phil nodded in agreement. "And my roommate Eric is a vegetarian as well."

"Wow," Rhonda said. "I'm not even a vegetarian."

"Then you're a murderer!" Phil screamed.

No, he didn't. Phil had grown up a lot by then. And so had Matt.

He passed that screening interview, and then he got the e-mail that would change everything.

Fourteen dogs had been surrendered from a puppy mill in Kentucky, and they needed fosters in the Midwest immediately. A foster family would usually care for a dog for somewhere between one to three months before a permanent family could be located.

A few days later, Matt, accompanied by his friend Ashley, pulled up next to a muddy red van in a McDonald's parking lot in Brighton, Michigan, to do his part. It was a gloomy, cold Sunday in October 2009. The proximity of the McDonald's no longer tempted Matt, though it did provide a funny juxtaposition. That parking lot, where he would be meeting a dog so he could volunteer his time and amp up the level of responsibility in his life, was also the site where, years before, he would skip out on Sunday school in order to avoid responsibility and expectations. But now Matt was a new man.

Jen, a generous and friendly volunteer for CRUSA, greeted us and gave some context and warning.

"Now, you really understand, this is more than just looking after a pet, you hear?"

"I understand," Matt said.

"These dogs were in conditions none of us could fathom. You have no idea how mistreated they may have been. They could have been beaten. Or starved. Or kept in a dark room for days at a time. He'll have to teach you what he can stand and what he can't. He might not be able to eat with you in the same room. He might not be able to have the door closed. Noises that you might not find disturbing could be terrifying for him."

"I'll do my best," Matt said. "I'm not looking for someone to fetch my slippers—I just want to help."

MR. PEYTERSON

Jen smiled and nodded. As she opened the side door and pulled out a tiny little crate, the stench of urine was overwhelming. Inside stood a tiny, shivering, salt-and-pepper cairn terrier fur ball, completely petrified. He was crusty and smelled horrible, but Matt didn't give a fuck. The four-month-old pup's name was Peyton, and Matt hugged that dude and got a little misty-eyed just thinking about all the pain and torment he and his compadres had already dealt with in just their brief welcome into the world.

It was something no one should ever deal with.

There's nothing more rewarding than putting your money where your mouth is, to actually do your part to address terrible things happening in the world. And this was one of those profound moments for Matt.

We brought Peyton home, immediately gave him a bath, and got acquainted. Matt went through the process of fostering: getting Peyton checked out at the vet, getting him neutered, etc. He felt a bond forming.

Peyton became his shadow. He loved riding in the car. He'd go to work with Matt. He'd go over to our parents' house for dinner on the weekends, and just about every-thing else.

Peyton was smart. Within a week or two, he had already learned to sit and shake hands. But the most adorable thing, which became his signature move, was when he popped up on his hind legs and hung out there staring at you trying to figure out what he wanted to do.

Needless to say, Matt quickly realized he was failing. As a foster, at least. He didn't just want to take care of Peyton until someone else was ready to adopt him. Matt wanted to adopt him himself.

After many conversations with Phil and our parents, discussing the responsibility and ramifications, Matt made the decision. Peyton was family.

PETS ARE MEAT (BUT WE LOVE THEM)

What the meat and dairy industries don't seem to realize is we (humans) have sleeping giants in our homes. People love their pets.

In the US alone, some statistics estimate over 50 percent of households have a pet. And this is just taking into account traditional pets like cats and dogs. If you factor in things like illegal alligators and ferrets, those numbers get even bigger.

Animal agriculture was successful for years at lulling to sleep the cognitive dissonance that rages inside of us. They've turned the meat on our plate and the milk in our glass into a simple product we buy at the grocery store. A commodity with no face, no name, and no feelings. A lie that keeps us petting our dogs and cats while eating their contemporaries. Mainly cows, pigs, chickens, and fish.

Have you noticed how as children we all show great awe and wonder at animals? Sure, some seem a little scary, but in general we all overwhelmingly care about animals and don't want them hurt.

But think about it. It's as though we're manipulated from an early age to think about animals differently. As less than. As objects. As food. And eventually we start to believe it more and more. As we grow up, we grow so disconnected from it, we forget. And then we start the cycle all over again with our kids.

What if kids are right and the parents are wrong? What if we're meant to care about animals and do all we can to protect them?

Matt realized there's a reason dogs are regarded as man's best friend. It's because he loves that little guy, and Matt is as devoted to him as Peyton is to Matt. It's man's best "friend," not man's best "accessory."

So love those little fur balls. Give them lots of pats and scratches and cuddles, because they deserve it. Just remember that if you like giving your parakeet a tickle under the chin, there's a chicken somewhere who'd probably appreciate it as well.

CHAPTER 5

CHAMPION AS FUCK: HOW TO BECOME THE GREATEST ATHLETE IN ALL OF HISTORY

CLEARLY WE LOVE OUR PETS. And we're fascinated by them. Matt's dog, Peyton, can be energetic, inquisitive, excitable, demanding, and a million other things that show him to have a dynamic personality with a depth of wants and needs. Just like a person.

But a few people still want to eat them (the animals, not the people).

And that makes sense, too, in a way. When Phil first expressed his interest in giving up meat, our dad was having none of that shit. Something he kept coming back to was "It's going to make you weak and sick." Our dad seemed to equate meat with muscle. Which, in some ways, is perfectly logical. When people eat meat, they are mostly eating the muscles of the animal (people only tend to eat things like the organs of an animal if they're eating at either a very fancy or a very not-fancy restaurant. And pretty soon it will only be at not-fancy restaurants. And soon after that it won't be available anywhere).

We're sure that, at some point thousands of years ago, a dude saw a deer running, saw those muscles rippling, saw the speed the deer possessed, the height it was able to jump so explosively and effortlessly, and thought, *I want to have that kind of power.*

> **FUN FACT:** Bambi's mom was a deer, and we all cried when she was shot and killed.

Then it wasn't much of a jump (no pun intended!) for that dude to conclude, "If I eat that creature, I will devour his strength, and then his power will become my power." And so the dude tracked that deer and killed him and ate him. And you know what? He probably did feel stronger. You know why? When you're living a hunter-gatherer existence, you're in a constant state of starvation, and eating *anything* is going to make you feel fucking stronger and better. Especially if you have to run twenty miles around the plains to kill a goddamn deer.

The same goes for lots of different animals that have

been hunted over the years. Trappers seeking bear had to imagine that consuming the bear's flesh might also imbue them with the bear's strength. Hunters going after buffalo must have believed that dining on their bodies meant they would also be ingesting the power of the two-thousand-pound beasts. Fish and birds are quick. Alligators are scary as shit. Snakes move like lightning. If you want to be strong and fast and powerful and dynamic, you just need to eat meat, right?

Wrong, bitches.

ABSOLUTE DOMINATION

Here's a little experiment. What if we ask you to think about the most powerful, most successful, most dominating female athlete of the last fifty years? Who would you think of?

Really, there's only one correct answer: Serena Williams. Let's look at the data.

She's won twenty-three grand slam singles titles, the second most of all time. She's also won sixteen grand slam doubles titles and four Olympic gold medals in singles and doubles. She has amassed over $81 million in prize money, the most ever. (Not to mention all of her millions upon millions in epic endorsement cash.) She is one of three players in the history of professional tennis to have won a career slam in both singles and doubles (and, with sister Venus, the only pair to win a career doubles golden slam by also winning Olympic gold). Her six US Open titles are the most in the open era. Her seven Australian Open titles are also a record for most wins in the open era. She is the only person in the history of tennis, male or female, to win three majors six times. She has won more grand slam singles matches—309—than any player, male or female, in tennis history.

She is incredible.

She is dynamic.

She is powerful.

Know what else?

She is vegan.

What?! The greatest female athlete in history is vegan? We shit you not.

For Serena, the move to a vegan diet started with her sister Venus. In 2011, Venus noticed feelings of tremendous fatigue. While it wasn't unusual for a professional athlete to tire after a match, this was something she couldn't seem to shake. She was eventually diagnosed with Sjögren's syndrome, an incurable (and unspellable) autoimmune disease. Basically, Venus's immune system began viewing her own body as a threat, and started attacking. Venus's own body was trying to kill her. In addition to medication, her doctors suggested Venus adopt a vegan diet, believing it would help reduce joint inflammation associated with Sjögren's.

Serena, determined to support her sister in a difficult time, followed suit and also became vegan.

Did going off meat mean that Serena lost her edge? That she could only watch helplessly as her power and speed abandoned her? Hell no. Since transitioning to a vegan diet in 2012, at the ripe old age of thirty-one (ancient for a professional tennis player), Serena has won the Australian Open twice, the French Open twice, Wimbledon three times, and the US Open three times. That's ten majors. If she never wins another title in her career, those ten majors alone would place her sixth on the all-time list for major singles titles in the open era. It's pretty fucking safe to say that eating vegan hasn't slowed Serena down.

She won thirteen titles in thirteen years with her old diet (averaging one title per year), and then ten titles in four years since transitioning to a vegan diet (averaging 2.5 titles per year). She's more than doubled the rate at which she's been winning, and doing it all after the age of thirty, when most tennis players are forced to retire. Martina Hingis won her final major at nineteen. Monica Seles was only twenty-three when she won her last one. John McEnroe won his last major title at twenty-five. Same with Björn Borg. Steffi Graf and Ivan Lendl's last big wins were at thirty. Rod Laver and Pete Sampras both caught their last title at thirty-one. Chris Evert's final major came at thirty-two.

Serena's most recent major victory was at thirty-six, and she's still the one to beat every time she takes the court.

How's that possible? Wouldn't she have lost her athleticism without the dynamic effects of meat? Wouldn't a diet of tofu and eggplant and fruit and nuts make her fragile and passive?

Apparently not. If anything, it seems that eating vegan made Serena, already historically great, even *more* dominant. Makes you wonder what she would have done in her career if she'd been vegan from the start! She'd probably have about thirty-five titles and have obliterated every record in professional tennis!

SPEED

"But wait," some weird people say. "Tennis is a game of strategy and finesse and technology. The elite players use braided carbon–and-Kevlar racquets that can fire a tennis ball through a brick wall all by themselves. Those elements help compensate for any requirement for EXPLOSIVE ATHLETICISM. Convince me you can be explosive without meat!"

Oh, okay. Perhaps we can introduce you to Carl Lewis?

Carl Lewis is one of the most decorated athletes in history. He won nine Olympic gold medals, eight world championships, and some victories in the Goodwill Games and Pan American Games. But damn! Nine Olympic gold medals!

FUN FACT: Humans, at their fastest, can run almost thirty mph. This makes them slower than just about everything in the animal kingdom that might want to eat them (cheetahs can go over seventy mph, lions around fifty mph, tigers at forty mph, wild dogs and coyotes at over forty mph, and hyenas at thirty-seven mph. So basically, humans are amazing. And animals are amazing, too.

When Lewis was approaching thirty, he knew that he was on the downward swing of his career. Most sprinters (like most tennis players, or most any athlete—sports are hard) peak in their early or midtwenties. Maurice Green saw his last gold medal at the ripe old age of twenty-six. FloJo was done by twenty-nine. Donovan Bailey's last gold came at thirty. In a sporting discipline that relies so heavily on raw athleticism, there are fewer opportunities for a veteran runner to improve his performance through strategy and guile. The gun sounds, you run as fast as you can, and you win or you lose. Unlike in football, you can't study hours of game film. Unlike basketball, you can't spend the summer adding a three-point shot or a low-post game. So when Carl Lewis felt that his athletic performance wasn't everything he wanted it to be, what did he do?

He transitioned to a vegan diet.

In 1990, Lewis decided that he would cut out meat and

dairy. The result? One of the greatest world championships of his stellar career, earning a gold in the 100 meters (setting a world record in the process), another in the 4×100-meter relay, and a silver medal in the long jump. Despite forgoing meat, Carl Lewis still proved to be one of the fastest, most dynamic athletes on the planet.

MAKE 'EM BLEED

"But wait!" you say. "Speed and strength aren't the same thing. Greyhounds are fast, but they're not powerful. Only by eating meat can you be powerful!"

To those people, I say two words: Nate Diaz.

When a lot of people think of a UFC power hitter, they think of someone like Nate Diaz. He is a powerful 20-11-0 fighter who beat the likes of Conor McGregor. Nate has stated about being vegan: "I hear a lot of criticism from people saying you need meat to be strong and for recovery, and it's a bunch of bullshit because I train harder than everybody. It's so easy to argue with these people. I'm like, 'Dude, have you done a tenth of what I've done?'"

Vegan eating has virtually taken over the UFC, as the list of fighters turning vegan just keeps on growing. Nate's brother Nick, Jake Shields, Mac Danzig, Matt Wiman, James Wilks, Ashlee Evans-Smith, Heather Jo Clark, and the list goes on. Not only are these athletes vegan, they're vegan in the most brutal and intense sport on the planet.

FOOTBALL

"But wait!" you say. "Who's ever heard of UFC anyway? What about some real American sports people watch on TV every weekend?"

First of all, that's bullshit. But you haven't had enough meatless power? How about Tony Gonzalez? Depending on how Rob Gronkowski's body holds up, Tony Gonzalez will go to the NFL Hall of Fame as the greatest tight end the game has ever seen. At six five and 247 pounds, Gonzalez is what many might charitably call "somewhat physically intimidating." He was a fourteen-time Pro Bowl selection. He holds every significant record for a tight end in professional football, including most touchdowns (111), most receiving yards (15,127), and most receptions (1,325).

Gonzalez was first turned on to vegetarianism when he shared a flight with a man named David Pulaski, who refused to eat the meat served to him at dinner. While it's true that most people refusing to eat airline food would be no surprise, this was first class. They were probably being served porterhouses and lobster, but Pulaski pushed it aside. He told Gonzalez about the health costs of consuming meat, even sharing with him the results of a study in China (if you're interested, check out *The China Study* by T. Colin Campbell and Thomas M. Campbell) that showed that people who ate the fewest animal products were the citizens most likely to avoid a wide variety of illnesses and ailments. Pulaski managed to do a convincing enough job that the tight end decided to become a vegetarian. Gonzalez experimented with different dietary approaches, at times being a strict vegan, other times being just a vegetarian, and other times still including some meat, eventually adopting an 80/20 approach to meat in his diet (80 percent plant-based foods and 20 percent meat). We'll go more into the semimeatless in Chapter 7.

MEATABETES

So professional athletes are going vegan in droves now. Is there any downside to a heavy meat diet?

This is not going to surprise anybody. Everyone has heard news reports about how consuming a lot of meat can lead to heart disease. But even more clear than that, most people have fried up a pound of beef to make tacos, and then drained off the fat into a coffee can. What did it look like? It looked like about a cup of grease that then hardens into yellow, waxy fat. That's not just going into the coffee can you're pouring it into—it's going into your body. So perhaps it's no surprise that researchers linked a compound in red meat called carnitine to atherosclerosis, or the hardening or clogging of arteries. They found that high levels of carnitine were also correlated with an increased risk for heart disease.

Makes sense. You take in more gloppy fat, it's going to

gum up your works. What else can it cause? How about diabetes?

"No way!" you say. "Diabetes is caused by eating candy bars and drinking Mountain Dew!" Well, the Mountain Dew won't help. But according to a study in *JAMA Internal Medicine*, eating just a few ounces of red meat or processed meat (hot dogs, bologna, salami, etc.) could increase your risk for type 2 diabetes by up to 50 percent. There are three components of meat that can contribute to diabetes, according to researchers at the Harvard School for Public Health (HSPH): sodium, nitrites, and iron. Sodium can cause insulin resistance. Nitrites also cause insulin resistance and can adversely affect the pancreas. Iron can cause damage to people who have a genetic predisposition for super iron absorption. The study found that swapping out meat for other foods, like whole grains, nuts, and other vegan-beloved chow, would significantly reduce a person's diabetes risk.

So just to review: eating vegan won't slow you down, but eating meat might actually lead to you getting your feet amputated. Which would slow you down.

MEAT HEADS (NOT WHAT YOU THINK)

You know what else eating meat can cause? Alzheimer's. UCLA had a study that showed that red meat has a shit-ton of iron, and increased consumption of iron can cause problems. There's this thing called myelin—it's sort of like varnish that covers your brain's neural fibers—and when you start getting a lot of iron in your brain, it breaks down the myelin, which can fuck up your brain communication, which can cause Alzheimer's-like symptoms. The more meat, the more iron; the more iron, the less myelin; and the less myelin, the worse your brain works. Meat literally can make your brain work like shit.

You know what else can end up suffering? Your junk.

According to the *American Journal of Cardiology* in an article titled, "The Link Between Erectile and Cardiovascular Health: The Canary in the Coal Mine," erectile dysfunction affects up to 30 million men in America, and 100 million men worldwide.

Hold on a second. Men in America make up only about 8 percent of men worldwide. Yet they make up 30 percent of the world ED population. WTF.

In a subsequent article in the *American Journal of Cardiology*, titled "The Artery Size Hypothesis: A Macrovascular Link Between Erectile Dysfunction and Coronary Artery Disease," the authors made the case that erectile dysfunction and coronary artery disease are different versions of the same disease.

The same arteries that get clogged from cholesterol are present in your junk. But guess what? Those arteries are even smaller.

Which means they get clogged a whole lot faster.

So men in America are suffering from limp-dick syndrome, and doctors are just giving them pills to jack up their blood flow. That treats the symptom, but not the cause.

So if you're having trouble in the sack, maybe change your diet before getting a prescription for new boner pills.

Your libido is suffering because meat is slowly killing you.

And then you're left wanting to have sex, but unable to perform.

Here we are again destroying that myth that meat makes you a man. Eating meat can actually make you *less* potent in bed.

Basically your penis is a window into your heart. And if you can't get it up, you're poised for some far more serious health issues down the road besides the obvious one—crying yourself to sleep every night alone in the fetal position.

Since a vegan diet is naturally higher in nutrients and lower in cholesterol, it's going to get you hard again, and keep you hard as you age.

You'll be the gigolo of the old folks' home.

But the even better news about this is when your sexual performance returns, so does your health. Your overall heart health will improve.

Now we've been pretty clear. We're not some of those snake-oil-salesman types. We're not making outrageous health claims and insinuating that vegan is the holy grail of health and you'll live young and beautiful for all of eternity.

We're merely giving you some balanced information that indicates that there may well be some health benefits that accompany your compassionate motives to eat vegan.

So heart disease, diabetes, Alzheimer's, erectile dysfunction—that's just some of the damage that meat can do to your body directly. You know what else can happen? It can make some shit hitch a ride.

E. COLI FOR PRESIDENT

One of those hitchhikers: E. coli.

This made national news a couple of decades ago. In 1993, 732 people were infected with E. coli bacteria that came from undercooked hamburgers served at the fast-food chain Jack in the Box. The majority of the victims were little kids, and four of them died. Of the other victims, 178 suffered serious and permanent health consequences, including impaired brain and kidney function. It was, arguably, the most notorious case of food poisoning in American history.

The E. coli–tainted meat caused what's called hemolytic uremic syndrome, or HUS. E. coli damages red blood cells, and the damaged red blood cells then clog the kidneys. With the kidneys all clogged up, the body starts to go into kidney failure. The kidneys help filter toxins from the blood, and with compromised kidneys, people with HUS then suffer from vomiting, bloody diarrhea, abdominal pain, headaches, and fevers and chills. As the condition progresses, people can suffer from edema (swelling of the legs), blood in the urine, sweating, and unexplained bruises. This can lead to complications such as seizures, heart problems, stroke, or coma. And even death.

And it all came from a contaminated hamburger.

> **WTF:** Check out *Fast Food Nation* for a description of how meat inspections work. Basically, there are almost no meat inspectors, and when the ones that exist want to do an inspection, they have to make an appointment with the place they're inspecting.

E. coli isn't the only thing to watch out for. Remember mad cow? Or as it's also known, BSE (bovine spongiform encephalopathy). This degenerative brain disease affected cows, primarily in Britain from the mid '80s to the late '90s. Cows suffering from BSE would show increased aggression, respond angrily to sounds or touch, refuse to eat, and show a profound loss of coordination, stumbling and falling about. It was fucking sad.

You know how that shit got started? Cows, who are normally herbivores, were given feed containing some meat (from either other cows or sheep), possibly as a strategy to bulk them up. When cows ingest brain or spinal cord material (or a bunch of other things) from other animals, it's not natural and shit can go wrong. That's how the cows were first exposed to BSE. Then it incubated for a while, up to five years, and it spread.

In the UK, they ended up finding almost two hundred thousand cows with BSE, and almost two hundred people died from the disease. You know how they put a stop to it? They basically killed a shit-ton of cows. They slaughtered 4.4 *million* cows to prevent further spread of the disease.

That's a goddamn tragedy. Do you think they have carrot spongiform encephalopathy? Or soybean spongiform encephalopathy? Hell no, they do not. Think about that the next time you're carving into a steak.

When humans ingest meat with BSE, they can develop Creutzfeldt-Jakob disease (CJD). Those who have the disease tend to show symptoms around the age of sixty, and then die about a year later. That shit's serious. When the disease first hits, those afflicted can suffer from memory loss, change in behavior, diminished coordination, and visual problems. As the condition progresses, sufferers can experience insomnia, depression, muscle spasms, blindness, weakness in the extremities, coma, and then death. It's no picnic, no pun intended.

THERE'S NO *I* IN TEAM, BUT THERE ARE HORMONES IN MEAT

Another thing that they like to add to meat: hormones. In their natural state, cows will eat grass. But you don't see rapid weight gain with grass, so ranchers often feed them other things (like feed tainted with animal proteins and BSE, as seen above), and they also inject them full of hormones to promote weight gain. And it's not like they somehow vacuum that shit up once they shoot a metal rod through the cow's forehead at slaughter. So people who eat meat consume those hormones as well. In a study published in the *Archives of American Medicine*, women who consumed more than six ounces of red meat a day were twice as likely to develop hormone-sensitive breast cancer as women who ate the same amount of meat every other day. Researchers speculate that the hormones may attach themselves to cancer cells and spur their growth.

CANCER, OSTEOPOROSIS, AND STONES

On the subject of cancer, a National Cancer Institute Study found that of five hundred thousand people sampled, people who ate meat every day had a 30 percent increased chance of dying over a ten-year period over people who ate the least amount of meat. As scientists are quick to say, correlation is not necessarily causation (they should just print that on a T-shirt), but it is a bit sobering.

Even when meat doesn't kill you or rot your brain or cause cancer, it still can have harsh effects on your health. For instance, eating meat has also been shown to increase the risk of osteoporosis. Meat and eggs are composed of sulfur-containing amino acids, and when we eat them, they metabolize as sulfuric acid. The body attempts to neutralize the acid by introducing calcium, and you know where that calcium comes from? Our bones. So we leach calcium out of our bones to help neutralize the acid, and then pee that down the toilet, along with our hopes and dreams. Researchers at the National Institutes of Health found that increased meat consumption could lead to lower amounts of bone formation, long-term decrease in bone density, and greater susceptibility to osteoporosis.

There has also been research showing a link between meat consumption and kidney stones and gallstones. Now, kidney and gallstones are no joke. These accumulations of minerals can be as small as a grain of sand or as large as a golf ball. Most of the time, people pass these stones out in urine, but can you imagine trying to force a golf ball–sized rock out of your cock? We've discussed it and concluded that the only thing that sounds more painful and uncomfortable would be to try to cram a golf ball–sized rock *into* your cock. And if you could minimize your risk of this by eating less meat, then shit yeah, that sounds like a pretty convincing argument. So, you know, if you're not into that sort of thing, then, well, you're already vegan at heart and groin. And if you are into that sort of thing, all we can say is, be safe! That type of fetish can be quite dangerous, and we doubt you want to end up in the emergency room telling a doctor how a rock got stuck in your urethra.

So maybe our dad was a little off base when he tried pushing meat onto our plates for fear that we'd get weaker and sicker. There's plenty of evidence to show this was a bunch of bullshit, the knee-jerk response of a man who'd been raised for decades to think, *Eat a strong animal and become a strong animal.*

And to top it off, meat can cause a number of terrible medical problems, from coronary disease to diabetes to impotence and kidney stones.

MY, WHAT A BEAUTIFUL CORPSE YOU HAVE

There's a quote, often incorrectly attributed to James Dean, that goes "Live fast, die young, leave a beautiful corpse." There are some people who would say, "Why should I worry about the health consequences of my food if we're all going to die anyway?" The reason being: BECAUSE DOESN'T THAT SEEM LIKE AN IDIOTIC WAY TO THINK?! If it's snowing outside, we put on our boots, because walking barefoot in the snow is going to burn our feet and make them uncomfortable. Even if we'll die someday, that doesn't mean that we WANT to experience as much pain as possible. Pain sucks. If you want to think, *Life is short, so fuck up your body and damn the consequences,* you can do that. But if you want to think, *Life is short, and enjoy the time you have, bro,* you can do that, too. Not having heart attacks feels good. Avoiding Alzheimer's feels good. Sex feels good. And if eating vegan will help in those departments, who would want to say no?

CHAPTER 6

EXPLODING SHIT LAKES: VEGANS AND THE ENVIRONMENT

CLEARLY, THERE ARE NO GOOD reasons to eat vegan. Better sex, fewer heart attacks, less mad cow disease, not being an asshole to animals, maybe less chance of contracting cancer, and Serena Williams winning championships. You know, no big deal at all.

So those are all ticks in the win column. But you know another reason eating vegan is stupid?

It helps everyone.

It's true! Eating vegan won't just clean up your heart, but it will also clean up land, water, and the air. And what kind of asshole wants clean land, water, and air?

How does it work?

WE FEEL WEIRD WRITING ABOUT FARTS (SORRY)

Vegan farts are pure magic. It's like having a genie in a bottle, but in your ass instead. Vegans release a gaseous ambrosia from their assholes that adds important nitrogen to the air and also emits an aroma that's kind of a blend of sandalwood and new-car smell.

Well, that's not actually true.

But seriously, motherfucker. Eating vegan does help.

Our decisions about how we eat affect literally BILLIONS of people. Because agribusiness makes a huge, corrosive impact on the environment.

Most people know that one of the biggest producers of greenhouse gases are the emissions made by burning fossil fuels for heat. Burning oil and natural gas produces a lot of CO_2. You know what else produces a lot of gas? Farts.

Seriously this time!

The UN says that the number one contributor of greenhouse gas emissions is agriculture. And most of that is from the methane produced by animals when they fart and shit. We shit you not (though the animals might). The average cow produces between 150–260 pounds of methane per year. That's almost as much as both of us combined! Or one Matt from his fat days!

Here's some more crazy shit: methane is messed up. Like the worst. And a lot of it (farts) comes out of cow butts. And the farts that come out of those cow butts?

Well, let's just say they're far worse on the environment than some of the other gases. Picture poison coming out of cow butts and floating into the air. Circulating all around, and ruining the party that we call life on this planet. Methane's effect on the environment is actually twenty-three times more jacked than CO2. Is that dangerous?

What are you? Some kind of asshole? Don't ever ask a stupid question like that! Just kidding. Asking questions is always a good thing. But this is some basic shit.

But guess what? As DJ Khaled would say, "They don't want you to know." The proverbial wool has been pulled over our eyes.

Who is "they"? Glad you asked. In this case, "they" is big agriculture. AKA the bullies who spend millions of dollars to keep all of us from learning these facts.

> **WTF:** According to opensecrets.org, agribusiness spent almost $60 million on campaign contributions to Congress in 2016, because "they" want to keep you in the dark, and they'll use any means necessary to mislead and lie to you.

"They" don't want us to learn these facts. So we're learning these fucking facts. And when more of us do, they will stop laughing all the way to the bank. And they will stop profiting hugely by fucking up the environment. And they will realize they have a choice: A) their money train will stop, or B) they'll make a ton of money doing something else.

Still, you might say they provide some benefit, in a sense. After all, they bring people together from all over the political spectrum. Why? Because everyone hates the shit they're doing. Oh, and also, supposedly, people really hate being lied to and manipulated like puppets.

But we digress.

SHIT LAKES

So, is methane dangerous? Yes, dude. That shit is dangerous! Just to give you some idea about the potency and lethality of methane, imagine a lake of pig shit. You don't even have to imagine it—just Google "feces lake." While we're sure that the fifth page of results is probably some pretty weird fetish site that would make us throw up in our mouths, the top results will be what was captured by a drone flying over a pig farm, and it's literally a lake of pig shit. These "lagoons," as they're called, can occupy over seven acres of land. They can hold up to 45 million gallons of urine, feces, and wastewater. That's enough to fill an Olympic-sized swimming pool in every one of the fifty states, and then have enough left over for *eighteen more*. Which makes sense, when you realize that a 180-pound pig, about the size of an adult American male, produces about eleven pounds of shit every day. These places literally smell like death—buzzards come flying in, thinking they've discovered the world's largest carcass.

Nope, it's not gross at all.

And it's not dangerous, either. There's a reason that your finer cafés and restaurants have signs saying "Employees Must Wash Hands." It's because that's what upstanding citizens do. And also possibly because poop carries disease. Now imagine an employee at a restaurant shitting one hundred times a day. And his five thousand coworkers (it's a huge restaurant, like a Cracker Barrel the size of an airplane hangar). And they never wash their hands. That sounds like a restaurant we would all love to eat at, doesn't it? No. No, it doesn't. So you can see there may be a few problems when it comes to working in an industrial pig, cow, or chicken farm.

BACTERIA ROULETTE

Have you ever heard of campylobacter? Neither had we. But as we uncovered the facts for this chapter we saw this word, and we thought to ourselves, *Let's find out what this damn word means.* Well, people working on chicken farms on the Delmarva Peninsula in Maryland actually know what this word means. It's a kind of bacteria you can find in chickens and chicken shit, and it can cause diarrhea and abdominal pain and can even be fatal. When examining three different groups for the disease, Dr. Ellen Silbergeld discovered that 41 percent of chicken wranglers tested positive for the bacteria, as did 63 percent of employees working inside the processing plant, and 100 percent of the town residents that were tested for the study. Holy fuck! According to a 2010 issue of *Consumer Reports*, 62 percent of all chicken sold at supermarkets have the bacteria. Most people wouldn't play Russian roulette, because there's a 17 percent chance that they'd have a bad outcome. And by "bad outcome," we mean death. But some crazy fuckers still eat chicken, when there's a 62 percent chance of consuming some disgusting bacteria? That's like playing Russian roulette with four bullets in the gun. Clearly, that's just brilliant game theory there. "There's only a one in three chance that eating this won't add some killer bacteria into my guts? I'm going to take seconds, bro! Excuse me, waiter? Give me more of that deadly chicken bacteria, please."

EVEN E. COLI EVOLVES

We have evolved. We created electricity and iPhones. But the bad news is that E. coli has evolved as well. E. coli is still out there, and it's also gotten tougher. Normally, cows eat grass, if left to their own bovine devices. But to make them fatter, factory farms feed them higher concentrations of grain, which has caused the acid in the cows' stomachs to become stronger in order to break that shit down. As a result, E. coli has evolved to survive the more acidic cow stomach. So basically, E. coli is getting better. Like E. coli is winning. The bad news is that when E. coli wins, we die.

In the past, humans weren't as susceptible to E. coli, because our stomach acid was more concentrated than that of the cows. But now that E. coli has evolved to live in the more inhospitable environment provided by the cows, it's more of a threat to people as well.

Nope, nothing to worry about here. Move along. Avert your eyes.

SUPERBUGS!

It's a bird! It's a plane! No, wait . . . It's a superbug! This is another issue that plagues the factory farm: superbugs. When you pack a bunch of pigs or chickens or cows very close together, it's not good for the animals. One result of the close quarters and the methane and CO_2 that the animals constantly ventilate is that the animals' immune systems become compromised, which means that the animals get sicker and die more, and that leads to smaller profits. What could they do to make the animals healthier? Could they give them more room to live and eat? Hell no! What dipshit would suggest such a crazy solution? As a workaround, the factory farms give their animals TONS of antibiotics (70 percent of the antibiotics used in the United States are used on animals that are raised to be our food) to help kill some of these bugs, your E. colis and your campylobacters. And this saves the lives of many of the animals. You know what else it does?

It makes the bacteria SUPER STRONG! Which we normally wouldn't have a problem with. I mean we're pro getting stronger. Unfortunately, in this scenario, the stronger the bacteria is, the weaker we are. So we're kind of opposed to it.

The bacteria evolve, and they do it fast. And that means that the meat industrial complex has produced some extremely tough, very dangerous bugs that are resistant to antibiotics!

But, hey, what's the worst that could happen? Probably just a few cases of the sniffles, right?

Ever hear of MRSA? When infected, a person first presents with a fairly innocuous-seeming rash. Then it progresses to giant, pus-filled boils. MRSA can also spread to vital organs and lead to sepsis. Sometimes, treatment requires incision and drainage, where doctors have to basically cut the infection out. According to a report in *The Week*, European studies show a "strong causal link" between pig farms and MRSA. And according to a 2007 report by the CDC, MRSA now accounts for more deaths than HIV/AIDS. Listen, we love MRSA as much as the next person, but we'd be doing you a disservice if we didn't share this with you.

So, of course, no real concern. Totally normal.

This is partly because MRSA, and other bacterial infections, have become so drug resistant. It's like all these bacteria are wearing fucking Kevlar body armor now.

One of the strongest antibiotics currently on the market, vancomycin, is becoming useless in treating these kinds of superbugs. Vancomycin was at one point called a "last defense," because modern medicine just hasn't developed anything stronger. Now that final defense offers almost no resistance. Thanks, factory farming! High five!

> **FUN FACT:** A day's worth of vancomycin will run you about $70.

So factory farms produce lots of deadly bacteria. But that's not all. They also produce deadly, toxic gases.

KILLER GASES FROM PIG ASSES

Let's get back to our feces lakes. Those things aren't just eyesores—those lakes are deadly. Since it's full of pig waste, that means pig urine and pig feces, and THAT means it's a lake full of ammonia, hydrogen sulfide, carbon dioxide, carbon monoxide, methane, and other chemicals that can literally *dissolve metal*. And please understand, our goal here isn't to make pigs self-conscious about their poop and piss. But we have to be honest, their poop and piss is a dangerous combo. Because of this chemical stew, workers at pig farms have complained about burning eyes and throats, difficulty breathing, nausea, vomiting, and a host of other problems, *just from breathing the air around places like that.* The pigs live in tiny, cramped huts where the air gets so thick with methane and CO_2 and other poisonous gases that the farms need to run industrial-sized circulating fans to help clear it. If the fans malfunction for any reason for any length of time, the pigs die from inhaling their own poisonous gases.

The people don't do much better.

In Oklahoma in 1992, a worker was repairing something at one of these feces lakes when he started to choke to death on the toxic fumes. Another worker saw what was going on and dived into the lake of shit to save him. They both died. In Michigan, a worker was repairing something on another one of these lagoons when the fumes got to him and he collapsed. His fifteen-year-old nephew saw his uncle take a header into the lake of shit and dived in to save him, only to lose consciousness. The worker's cousin, older brother, and father were all nearby and tried to help save their fallen family, and all five of them died. We're not making this up. That really happened. THEY DIED just from being on a factory farm. Holy balls. That shit is serious.

Sounds like pretty safe working conditions. Probably has the same rate of days lost to injury or death as a Pottery Barn.

But we haven't even gotten to the coup de grace: exploding shit.

SHIT BOMBS

Around 2009, workers at pig farms observed what appeared to be a foam coating, a few feet thick, on the top of these feces lakes. Methane and other gases, instead of floating into the respiratory systems of unsuspecting workers, would instead get trapped under the foam. This created a huge risk if someone, say a casual smoker, were to put an open flame near these pits. Which happens. A lot. Hell, if you worked on a farm that smelled like a combination of sewer and three-day-old battlefield, you'd find ways to distract your sense of smell, too, we suppose. Just since 2009, there have been over thirty explosions around such sites, which have led to injured workers, exploding barns, and animals killed. In one incident like this, in Iowa, a methane blast killed 1,500 pigs. So you get an idea of how deadly and toxic these gases can be.

LOTF: LIFE OUTSIDE THE FARM

While dead workers and dead animals is horrible and tragic, the havoc that these deadly chemicals unleash affects an even wider group of victims. Even when those who suffer from airborne poisoning survive their encounters, it's still catastrophic. The *New York Times* ran a story about Robert Thornell, who was a neighbor near a factory farm. He wasn't a plumbing specialist whose work required him to swim in these shit lakes. He wasn't even a worker on the pig farm, which would require that he work in close proximity to the toxic ooze. He was just a regular guy who happened to live next to one of these farms. And it cost him dearly.

After living next to the factory farm for years, Thornell and his wife, Diane, started developing symptoms. They weren't sure what was happening to them. What was happening was that they were getting fucking brain damage. Just taking a breath near one of these shit farms was like taking a helmet-to-helmet hit from J. J. Watt.

Robert Thornell was the first to show the effects of toxic exposure. He was a schoolteacher, but can no longer work. He couldn't understand what was wrong with him, and worried that he'd had a nervous breakdown. Two years after first showing symptoms, he was diagnosed with irreversible brain injuries as a result of exposure to hydrogen sulfide gas. The former teacher used to be an animated talker with a quick smile, but now speaks slowly and forgets what he was talking about. He becomes so confused and disoriented that he can no longer travel any significant distance from his home for fear of becoming lost. The Thornells were told by their doctor to move, that while the effects of inhaling the nitrogen sulfide are irreversible, they can at least avoid future exposure and increasingly catastrophic symptoms. But Robert Thornell wasn't sure he'd be able to even sell his house. Besides, he'd already lived most of his life, over four decades, in that home, and didn't know how to move on.

Hey, if he didn't want to get permanent brain damage, he shouldn't have insisted on breathing all the time, right? Yes, that's actually sort of true. He did decide to live near a factory farm. But also, maybe, just maybe those fumes shouldn't really exist to begin with.

It's not just the Thornells. Other neighbors living next to factory farms have complained of chronic headaches, nosebleeds, fatigue, dizziness, memory loss, diarrhea, earaches, and lung burns. A joint study by the University of Iowa and Iowa State University found that up to 70 percent of factory farm workers suffer from acute bronchitis. The national average for that condition: less than 5 percent! You can't make this shit up, people.

Some people lose their sense of balance. Some report lack of sensation in their extremities. Can you imagine living next to a place so toxic that you lose sensation in your fingertips? Can you imagine having a son or a daughter who can't play baseball or football because they can't feel the ball when they try to throw it? You don't have to imagine it—just move next to an industrial meat farm, and you can live that fantasy.

The people who suffer from this poisoning have to buy nebulizers and supplemental oxygen tanks. But the oxygen tanks won't cure the damage—they'll only help reduce the symptoms. There is no cure. After being exposed to these poisons, the victims have to carry them and wheel them around for the rest of their lives.

DON'T DRINK THE WATER

The damage from pig farms isn't limited to the poisons they release in the air. They also contaminate the water. This occurred tragically in LaGrange County, Indiana, when the CDC was called in to investigate after a string of bad health outcomes. One woman had suffered four miscarriages without an obvious root cause. While examining this case, investigators discovered a neighbor of the first patient, living only half a mile away, who had also experienced a miscarriage, at approximately the same stage of gestation. While looking into this second case, a third case was discovered, only one mile away: a twenty-year-old woman who'd experienced a miscarriage at about the same gestational stage.

Investigators couldn't identify a genetic component for why these women would have been unable to carry their fetuses to term. Since they ruled out genetics as the reason for the miscarriages, they sought to test environmental causes. One clue they had was that a pig farm located in the area had been found years before to be a site of nitrate-contaminated drinking water. The maximum contaminant level for nitrates is 10 mg/L, but the water from the pig farm showed nitrate levels of over 50mg/L. Investigators decided to test the area's drinking water for heavy metals, bacteria, pesticides, and other poisons and contaminants.

They discovered only a single contaminant: nitrate.

For women in the town who had recently given birth to healthy babies, their water tested at an average of 3 mg/L. But the three women who experienced miscarriages? The nitrate levels in their water averaged over 20 mg/L, or almost *seven times* the levels of their healthy neighbors. After the initial cluster of women was studied, a fourth woman also suffered a miscarriage not far away. Her drinking water also showed dangerously high levels of nitrates.

The chemicals from the pig farm had poisoned the water, and then it poisoned the people in the town. Which I'm sure the pig farm would spin as a real positive. You know, keeps the price of rentals nice and low, no overcrowding at the playgrounds, shit like that. Fucking suburb of the year.

While the damage had been done, at least discovering the source of the problem meant that the residents could develop a solution to it. They stopped drinking the contaminated water. Instead, they began drinking bottled water or some form of treated water, and each of them, after making the switch, would later give birth to at least one healthy, full-term baby.

BLUE BABIES

In some respects, these women were lucky. But not every mother living near a factory farm will be able to rely upon an investigator to let her know if her drinking water is contaminated. For those who don't receive that kind of medical and scientific aid, they can run the risk of "blue baby" syndrome. A joint study by the U.S. Geological Survey and the Oklahoma Department of Agriculture found that ingesting water contaminated with nitrates over 10mg/L can lead to this condition, where the blood stops being able to carry oxygen as it normally would. Oxygen is what gives blood its red color, but when the blood is oxygen-depleted, the color of the blood changes, and the baby will appear to have a blue tinge. That baby is not getting enough oxygen. Blue baby syndrome can lead to a multitude of horrible medical consequences, such as increased rates of stomach cancer, birth defects, miscarriages, leukemia, and non-Hodgkin's lymphoma.

But if you're kind of psyched by the idea of your kid standing out in the crowd and think a blue baby would make you a celebrity mom, then this would actually be a real opportunity, right?

The meat industry doesn't just kill animals. It poisons the air, it poisons the water, and it kills people. You just have to admire their consistency.

GETTING A LITTLE GASSY (WE FEEL WEIRD AGAIN)

Another thing that you have to consider when you think about the impact of agriculture is that the seventh biggest contributor to greenhouse gas emissions is deforestation (which experts say contributes somewhere between 5–20 percent of greenhouse gas emissions). You know what takes in CO2 and converts it into oxygen? Plants. And big trees do a good job of scrubbing out that CO2. So when someone cuts down a tree, that CO2-scrubbing resource just goes away. Certainly, some of those trees are used to produce paper and shit (yeah, tons of people are using paper—when was the last time you got a letter? Ninety percent of paper goods are birthday cards wrapped around $5 checks sent by grandmothers to their grandkids who'll never write a thank-you note), but a lot of that deforestation is done as a way to create more pastureland for animals.

INEFFICIENCY EXPERTS: THE RIGHT WAY TO DO IT WRONG

Why is it that animals produce so many greenhouse gas emissions? Part of it is that making steaks and burgers is tremendously inefficient. Think about it. If you're trying to develop the ground beef for a burger, first you have to raise a cow. You start with a baby cow, and, assuming that that adorable baby cow isn't killed within his first six months to make an adorable veal, you feed him to fatten him up. You feed him grass and grain and sometimes the neural matter of other animals full of mad cow, and that helps make him bigger and fatter and marbled. The bigger he gets, the more shit he produces. That's got to go somewhere. More on that later. Then you slaughter him, putting his tougher cuts through a meat grinder to make ground beef, augmented in part by pink slime, this nasty fucking filler that's treated with ammonia. There! And we're supposed to enjoy those things we call burgers?!

But wait—why did you take all that grain and grass and feed it to the cow just to kill the cow to make dinner? Why didn't you just eat the fucking grain?! That's why it's so inefficient! You're basically processing your veggies through a cow to get something to eat, when you could just eat the veggies. That's kind of fucked up. It's sort of like converting all your paper money to coins, paying a 20 percent fee for the service, and then buying a six-pack and chips with the change. Who the hell would do that when you could just buy it in one easy step? Not you. You're smart.

David Pimentel, a professor of ecology at Cornell's College of Agricultural and Life Sciences, revealed some interesting numbers on how inefficient it all is. He noted that far more energy goes into meat production than it actually delivers. Beef requires about *fifty-four times* as much energy of input as one yields in protein output.

Gotta love that efficiency.

In an article he wrote for *TIME*, Bryan Walsh noted

that the beef industry is notoriously bad at getting the most yield from their product. In the United States, a cow consumes from seventy-five to three hundred pounds of grass or grain to produce a single pound of protein. In places like Africa that don't have quite the same level of quality of feed, the number can be as high as two thousand pounds to one. Literally a ton of grass and grain for every pound of meat produced!

Can you imagine if we did that for everything we consumed? Can you picture a dude feeding a goose gallons and gallons of water, just so that, two years later, when that goose is big and fat, he can then give him paper cuts and kick him in the balls until the goose cries from the abuse, and he drinks the tears? Of course he wouldn't—he'd just drink the water rather than go through the process of hydrating another animal just to consume his byproducts. So why is it so different with cows? Just eat the veggies and grains, dude.

> **FUN FACT:** We don't know what it is, but sometimes certain people just seem turned on by making things a lot more complicated, and a little more cruel.

WATER AND PEPSI

One of the most useful metrics to identify this inefficiency of resources is to look at the amount of water used to create different kinds of foodstuffs. Water is going to be a big deal in the future. In 2013, Pepsi CEO Peter Brabeck-Letmathe sent shock waves through the world when he said that some people believe that "as a human being you should have a right to water. That's an extreme solution." Brabeck-Letmathe seemed to argue that water should be controlled by people who could monetize it. Water scarcity will continue to drive people to attempt to own or control water rights and water supplies. If water is becoming increasingly valuable, how should that valuable resource be best put to use? Maybe *not* through fucking factory farming.

According to the *Huffington Post,* via the Water Footprint Network, in order to produce a single pound of beef, the beef industry has to pump in about 1,800 gallons of water. Compare that to how much water is used to produce one pound of that cow's favorite meals, corn: 147 gallons. It takes over *ten times* as much water to make a pound of beef than a pound of a vegetable.

That's a lot of water.

But maybe we're just using corn because it's the camel of vegetables. Let's look at some others. How about our beloved tofu? It's more demanding than corn, at about 300 gallons per pound (GPP), but nowhere near what beef requires. Though the soybeans themselves only require about 257 GPP. Potatoes are pretty easy, at 34 GPP. Oats are about 290.

How about fruit? On the low end, you have tomatoes,

at 26 GPP, then eggplant at about 43 GPP, then strawberries, pineapples, and watermelon, which require about 50 GPP. Oranges are about 67 GPP, grapefruit are 61, and lemons are 77. Apples, bananas, grapes, kiwis, and peaches are about 100 GPP. Avocados, though you might think are a vegetable because they're green, still have a pit, which is a seed (this will probably win you a pub quiz championship some night, so you're welcome), and they ring in at 140 GPP, still less than a tenth of what beef requires.

How about some vegetables? Broccoli, cauliflower, and Brussels sprouts are about 34 GPP. Which is good news for most people, with the exception of former president George H. W. Bush, who famously, and kind of bizarrely, said "I'm president of the United States, and I'm not going to eat any more broccoli!" It wasn't exactly the Gettysburg Address, but to each his own.

So basically, meat requires a shit-ton of water. But fruits and veggies, not so much. Shit, it takes six times as much water, per pound, as it does to produce tofu. Having a meat-heavy diet just demands more resources than a vegan diet.

NAUGHTY WATER

So that's the cost of water going into the agribusiness equation. What about the cost of water coming out? Or, more precisely, how much water is polluted, contaminated, poisoned, or otherwise destroyed by the meat industry?

We've already talked about some individuals who suffered as a result of contaminated water, but the craziest shit about this is it isn't just a few individuals who suffer—it's entire regions, THOUSANDS of square miles of land and water that are poisoned. You basically have to laugh so you don't cry.

Remember those feces lakes? Hard to forget, we know. How do you think they're formed? If you're like us, you imagine something like this: the pork (or beef or whatever meat is doing the shitting) plantation owner digs a HUGE hole, then someone pours concrete into the hole to create a barrier, like one would if he's preparing a nuclear power plant or some other hazardous waste risk. Then once those lagoons are filled, they are either treated to help make them less toxic before being recycled in some way (like human waste is), or drained and transported to an acceptable dumping site, or encased in more concrete and then sunk to the bottom of the ocean, like one does with spent nuclear rods. Or shot into the sun on a rocket called "The Vomit Comet."

FUN FACT: Matt and Phil are disgusted when people talk about vomit. And they apologize for doing it just now.

Think that's what happens?

That's not what happens.

They dig these shit pits, these lagoons, about thirty feet

deep. You know what they place at the bottom of it to stop the waste from seeping into the ground? Sometimes they use polyethylene liners. These work fine, unless there are rocks or metal cans or some other shit at the bottom that can tear into the liners, and when that happens, shit literally just seeps out. And that's for when they actually line it with something. Sometimes they don't. Then it just corrodes its way into the water table. You go to a home near a pig farm and turn on the tap, the water's going to smell faintly of shit.

Chicken, pork, and beef producers have to do something with the shit they produce, and a lot of them either accidentally or purposefully dump it in the nearest river or lake. The chemical reaction that takes place robs the waterway of its oxygen content, increases algae blooms (which also sucks up a bunch of the remaining oxygen), and kills fish through asphyxiation. In 1995, in North Carolina, a lagoon the size of *two football fields* ruptured, and 25 million gallons of pig shit flowed into the New River. The introduction of what was basically radioactive waste killed about 10 *million* fish. And that isn't an isolated incident. There are "dead zones" around the country where runoff from factory farms has proven so damaging and toxic that no aquatic life can survive. The largest of these dead zones is in the Gulf of Mexico, and is about the size of New Jersey (seems an appropriate state of comparison for chemical pollution).

Chesapeake Bay has also suffered greatly from the effects of factory farming. Perdue has a few chicken concerns in the area, to the tune of about 568 million chickens on the Delmarva Peninsula. That many chickens produce a ton of chicken shit, like over a billion pounds every year. A billion pounds of shit! That's 500,000 tons! Just for scale, the Empire State Building weighs about 365,000 tons, and a Nimitz-class aircraft carrier weighs about 100,000 tons, so just add those two together, and you're still about 35,000 tons short of the amount of weight equal to that much chicken shit. As a result of the chicken shit being introduced into the bay, Chesapeake Bay now only has about 12 percent of its volume with enough oxygen for the summer months.

And this kind of shit (literally) happens all the time. When Hurricane Floyd hit the East Coast in 1999, it slammed into these feces lakes like, well, a hurricane. And it's not like these lakes are in lockdown or are wrapped in Mylar envelopes or anything—they're just wide-open and brimming to the top. So when the hurricane hits, it just picks up all that shit and spreads it all over the state. Beaches miles from the feces lake ended up painted in pig shit.

And these places aren't just vulnerable to hurricanes. Since many of these lagoons are just open-air lakes of shit, they can overflow by something as simple and innocuous and common as a light rain. Or sometimes they overflow when a gas pocket forms underneath a lagoon using one of the liners, a ball of methane and ammonia growing and growing until it pushes all that toxic sludge over the edge.

How bad is it? As a polluter, agribusiness is in some ways worse than chemical or oil companies. For instance, Tyson (who produce a shitload of chickens) has to notify the EPA about pollution of their processing plants (which is not the sum total of their pollution, but whatever). Between 2010 and 2014, they dumped 104 *million tons* of pollutants into U.S. waterways. Think about that shit.

This is all to say that agribusiness isn't great for the environment. Many might say it's cruel, it's inefficient, it poisons the water, it poisons the land, and it contributes to global climate change. It's hard for one person to change the world, but one person can at least contribute to one part of it. There are advances being made, sure. *Popular Mechanics* recently published an article about how scientists accidentally discovered a process that would convert CO_2 into ethanol. And that's great, no question about it. But a couple of things: 1) this was a discovery made by accident, which means that the scientific community can't exactly pencil in a new world-changing innovation every six months, and 2) while we applaud the work of these scientists, we're doers. We like to do things. We like to contribute. We like to do our share. And just hoping that someone else can fix a problem seems like the height of laziness and irresponsibility. We do what we can to make the world a better place, and one of the things we can do is not eat meat.

So even if you don't care about the heart attacks, or erectile dysfunction, or mad cow, there's still the rest of the world out there, and that means you can still do something that will help everyone around you. And who wouldn't want to save the world? Other than most James Bond villains. But we have faith that the world is full of more people wanting to fix things than people trying to blow it all up.

CHAPTER 7

BADASS HOMEWORK: THE VEGAN PLAN OF ACTION

So you think trying vegan might be for you? You've thought about how eating meat hurts the animals, how it hurts the environment, and how it generally makes the world a worse place to be.

So what's next? Are you ready to move toward a vegan diet?

You literally just ate a hamburger yesterday. You can't possibly be vegan.

Well, we're here to say, "Yes, you can."

You can claim you're not vegan all you want, but face the facts. You are.

Some people take exception to that.

THE ARGUMENTS WE USED TO ENCOUNTER A LOT WHEN SOCIETY DIDN'T KNOW ANYTHING ABOUT A VEGAN DIET

There are a lot of people who haven't yet accepted the vegan inside of them. Some of those people offer arguments against it. Here's a sampling of some of the more convincing arguments that we run into in the course of our lives.

We're Apex Predators, Dude

Recently, we were approached by a somewhat animated dude at the dog park. We suspect that he was summoned by our conversation, debating whether we should have Beyond Meat tacos or some righteous Szechuan noodles with tofu for lunch. The dude, a man named Scooter (his name has not been changed to conceal his identity), seemed offended at our rejection of meat and insisted that humans should eat whatever they please because, as he reasoned, "We're at the top of the food chain."

As he said this, he reached down to pet his dog, a tiny little puffball of a Pomeranian. He was really cute (the dog we mean, though we guess Scooter was okay, too). And Matt said to Scooter, "Wow. You know what? You're right. So how about we eat your dog?"

Scooter blanched. "That's my best friend!" he said.

Phil grinned and replied, "But we're at the top of the food chain, big guy."

And then we ate his dog.

(Only the last part is an exaggeration.)

This is an argument we run into a lot. Some people seem to think that because we're the alphas on planet Earth, that this entitles us to do whatever we want. And in a way, those people are actually correct. But if it's okay to eat chickens or cows because we're so successful, then why is it wrong to eat dogs or cats? It's not like dogs are building their own cities or cats are inventing iPods. If being able to domesticate animals means that we can eat them, then it's as right, or as wrong, to eat a cat or a dog or a parrot or a gerbil as it would be to eat a cow or a pig.

Other people have argued that it's all about intelligence, that dogs are smarter than cows, and so we can spare the dogs and eat the cows. But pigs are smarter than dogs, and we eat them. Squid are also very intelligent, but we eat them. Ever hear of Inky? He's an octopus who escaped from the National Aquarium of New Zealand by climbing up his tank, squeezing through a narrow opening, slithering down the floor of the building, and then managing to enter a six-inch drainpipe that led to the sea. That's some straight-up Houdini shit, and people still eat octopus. And the world is FULL of total idiots, and we rarely eat them.

If Someone Else Does a Thing, I Can Do a Thing

A few weeks after our conversation with Scooter at the dog park, we were at the bookstore where Matt was buying *¡Salud! Vegan Mexican Cookbook*, by our good friend Eddie Garza. We encountered a woman named Bertha. She noticed Matt's book and decided her opinion was necessary, arguing that there was nothing wrong with eating meat. She made a really good point and almost got us, noting, "Animals eat other animals in the wild. So humans should do it, too." We were baffled that we hadn't realized that before.

But as we were on our way to Outback Steakhouse, ready to order a couple of dingo burgers, we got to thinking. And well, animals do lots of things we wouldn't or shouldn't do. Animals also sometimes rape other animals, eat their own young, and smell and eat one another's shit. Very rarely do you hear someone say, "Well, if an animal does it, then it's probably all right." If that were the case, people would jerk off in public (monkeys), enslave their own people (meerkats), and kidnap and abandon neighboring children (emperor penguins). After all, animals do it!

Another point to consider is that animals do eat other animals, but they rarely factory farm other animals. And they seem incapable of harvesting soybeans or having a digestive system that can support a vegetarian diet. So in some small, some would say trivial ways, there are slight differences between humans and other animals. Also, we can use the Internet.

So we ended up deciding against the dingo burgers at Outback. But we're still not sure if it was the right decision.

We'll be honest, though. There is one argument that has a really good point. "What's the argument?" you ask?

Plants Are People, Too

"But plants feel pain, too." Yes, that's right. We still don't have an answer to this one because slitting a cow's throat and watching her bleed out alive is exactly the same as mowing your fucking lawn.

Do you get the point?

Here's the thing. We love people who still eat meat. Many of you are our friends. But you say a lot of ill-informed shit sometimes: "We're at the top of the food chain." "Animals don't feel pain." "Lions eat other animals in the wild, so we should, too." "Animals were put here for us to eat." "Children are starving." "If we stop eating meat, cows will take over the world." Et-fucking-cetera.

And to be honest, we used to say the same things. But it's weird when you think about it—whenever we list reasons for eating animals, many of us seem to always conveniently leave out the animals that we love: dogs (and, fine, cats, too).

Think about that. Change those statements above, but include "dogs" in them. "We're at the top of the food chain, so we should eat dogs." "Dogs don't feel pain." "Dogs were put here for us to eat." "If we stop eating dogs, they'll take over the world."

There are lots of reasons not to go vegan. Lots of arguments against it. The thing is, we just haven't encountered a lot of *good* arguments against it. "My grandfather ate meat every day." Yeah, and he also used to get polio. Things change and evolve and get better. Roll with it. "We need to thin the herd." We're just not worried about a chicken population explosion destroying the world. "Hunting is how I bond with my dad." We have a lot of friends who used to bond with their dad while hunting. But as they got older they realized it's possible to bond without killing someone, even in Texas. Point being—anyone can make an argument, but we haven't met anyone who could voice the "we need to eat meat" position and actually get us to eat meat again.

So feel free to eat vegan. Here's how.

FIND WHAT WORKS BEST FOR YOU

For many people, it's something that takes time. And some may not even feel comfortable making the goal of hitting that 100 percent mark. It's completely up to you how far you take it.

One of the concepts we are best known for is the notion that eating vegan is not this all-or-nothing thing. Lots of people see everything as either you're all in or all out. That's some straight-up bullshit!

There's a lot of middle ground. Think about it. Think about how often you eat meat right now. What about just veganizing one of those meals? Or eat vegan meals half the week? Or even one day per week! You could do that.

Or hell, you could even eat vegan except for social events. You could eat vegan except for one meal per year. You could eat vegan except when you're at a wedding and the cake isn't vegan.

> **FUN FACT:** You know what makes a vegan wedding cake sweet? Sugar. The same thing that makes a nonvegan wedding cake sweet.

There is so much middle ground it's insane. But somehow it became this black-and-white, hypercompetitive, overlabeled thing, with crazy people screaming, "Shit or get off the pot!" Well, we're here to put a stop to that. And the people who would be screaming at you to shit or get off the pot will likely be too distracted yelling at us because they think we're watering down the definition of the word "vegan" (and we are). So you can thank us for taking the brunt of their tiny but vocal aggression. Seriously, these people will literally show up to our talks, interrupt us, and start screaming, "You're not vegan." It's hilarious, and we love it.

You have our permission to move forward as much or as little as you feel comfortable.

In an earlier chapter about athletes, we'd discussed Tony Gonzalez. Tony experimented with going total vegan, and eventually adopted a diet that dramatically reduced most of his meat consumption but didn't ban it 100 percent. And you know what? We applaud him for cutting lots of meat out of his diet! That's awesome! It doesn't have to be all or nothing.

VACATE THE COMFORT ZONE

Still, we do encourage you to take a step out of your comfort zone. Set a goal that makes you a tad uncomfortable but still seems 100 percent doable.

Once you've done that enough to feel confident moving forward, take another step. You can take as many or as few steps as you want. It's completely up to you.

But we do want to caution you from committing to eat vegan 100 percent of the time overnight. Yes, it has been done. But many times when someone does that, they can stay strong for a while, but one week or one month later they cave and go back to eating a shit-ton of meat. And they feel terrible about themselves.

It doesn't have to be that way, dude. Ease into it. Explore the food. Figure out what you can eat, what foods you like to eat, what foods you don't like, etc. In time, eating vegan will become second nature. But in the beginning it will take some effort.

The animals are counting on you. Don't fuck this shit up for the long-term.

And if you ever make a mistake, it's not the end of the fucking world. We all make mistakes. For instance, Phil used to be under the impression that spring rolls only had vegetables in them.

> **FUN FACT:** Phil loves the hell out of spring rolls.

We've already established that Phil is a moron. Recently he took a few bites of a spring roll and realized he'd been eating pork. Did it throw him for a loop? Yes. Does he feel bad about it? No. He learned something new that day, and now always asks if there's meat in the spring rolls. He didn't do anything wrong and tries his best to be a good vegan. He didn't scream, "Damn, I've besmirched my vegan virginity and now I can never be pure again!" He realized he'd made a mistake, he corrected it, and moved on. Being a good vegan means you help animals and people by how you eat—it doesn't mean that every day you score a 1600 on your vegan SATs.

We both ate meat for a long time. There's nothing we can do about the animals that suffered in the past as a result. But we can work to change it in the future. Still, there will be times when the restaurant screws up, or a product is mislabeled, or, hell, you just accidentally stick something in your mouth without thinking. It's okay. You got this. You're doing something amazing. Be proud of making the world a better place.

Our culture doesn't do process well. Our culture does all or nothing. It's hard to understand process. It's easy to understand absolutes. And as a result, people think that the only right way to be vegan is to never eat anything involved with animals. And if you do, then you're a failure who can never be a true vegan. And you know who gets turned off by this bullshit? Almost fucking everyone. You tell someone who eats meat seven days a week that they have to quit it forever or they're some total fuckup? That dude will either fail and never try again, or he'll never even make the attempt in the first place.

That's not what we're talking about.

LABEL YOURSELF WHATEVER YOU WANT

And, hell, if you don't even want to describe yourself as a vegan, don't. Who gives a shit what label you give yourself? You describe yourself however the hell you want. Vegan, plant-based, someone who doesn't eat meat, nothing, a piece of shit, the greatest human to ever walk the earth, whatever. And if someone gives you shit, just flip a table over and throw something at them.

No, don't actually do that. Just say something like, "Okay." Then walk away and laugh.

Now that labels are out of the way, think about your next step.

First of all, take a moment to think about everything you already eat that's vegan: fruit, vegetables, bread, nuts, Sour Patch Kids! *Sure*, you might be thinking, *but what about meat? I eat a lot of meat. And I could never give that up.* We're here to say that you don't have to—at least not all at once. Vegan eating isn't an all-or-nothing proposition. I guess what we're saying is: don't go cold turkey on the cold turkey. Do whatever makes you feel comfortable. But did you ever meet someone who ran a marathon? Did any of them train for it by showing up to the start line on marathon day and running 26.2 miles? Hell no! You got to train up to that shit!

> **FUN FACT:** Marathons seem really hard and neither of us have ever run more than a few miles. So we think it's pretty cool when people do that.

Anyone who tells you eating chicken three times a week is just as bad as eating chicken seven times a week is full of shit. We applaud the person who cuts meat down from seven meals to three. You have to start somewhere. Our mantra is: every meal makes a difference.

Some people eat vegan all year except for Thanksgiving dinner. And that's cool. We actually have a hack that has worked on many of our friends where we suggest that they only eat vegan on Thanksgiving and eat meat the rest of the year. After all, anyone can go one day without meat, even if it's National Turkey Day. We've found that people have so much fun veganizing their Thanksgiving dinner with us, and realize it's not all that hard, that they decide to eat vegan year-round, too. The point is, any step in the right direction is progress.

Besides, in today's world, it's impossible to be 100 percent perfect. Matt Ball, a vegan activist who heavily influenced us, writes: "The production of honey kills some insects, but so does driving (and sometimes even walking). Many soaps contain stearates, but the tires on cars and bicycles contain similar animal products. Some sugar is processed with bone char, but so is much municipal water." Does this mean that we have to stop using soap, or stop eating honey or sugar or drinking fucking tap water? Hell no! In other words: the goal of vegan eating isn't to be perfect. It's to do your best not to support animal abuse.

So let's take a step back and ask the crucial question: What ingredients cause the most suffering at the hands of factory farms? Meat. Fish. Dairy. Eggs. Simply avoiding these foods means you've already stopped supporting the vast majority of animal cruelty.

AVOID THE MINUTIAE

The problem is, sometimes it's easy to get sidetracked. There are a bunch of what-not-to-eat lists on the Internet and even a book titled *Animal Ingredients A-Z*. Do not look at this book or anything like it. Turns out there are a lot of things that may or may not have animal products in them. We encourage you not to give a shit about them. Don't get bogged down in the minutiae. Focus on the big picture. The foods that may or may not have animal products in them cause such a small amount of suffering that it's just not worth it. After all, what's better: trying to end 100 percent of all suffering but giving up after two weeks, or not worrying about that last .02 percent, but sticking with it for life?

The answer should be obvious. Don't become an ingredient nazi. By being douchebags, ingredient nazis turn other people off to vegan eating, which does more harm than good.

The reality is, being vegan is pretty simple. Don't make it harder than it has to be. For instance, some beer isn't technically vegan. Feel free to drink it anyway. The reason why not all beer is vegan is that some of it is processed with something called isinglass, which comes from fish bladders.

When a small percentage of beer is brewed, small particles of yeast may remain, so brew masters add a little bit of isinglass to the mix. This material then attaches to the yeast, congeals into a kind of gelatin, and sinks to the bottom of the beer cask, where it's isolated and thrown out.

> **FUN FACT:** Beer is delicious.

So that sounds disgusting. But the vast majority of fish aren't killed for isinglass, they're killed for people to eat. So if we stop eating fish but keep drinking beer, fish overall come out ahead. Therefore, by our calculations, practically all beer is vegan.

Brass tacks: if the food is not—or does not have in it—any of the "big-ticket" items of meat, fish, dairy, or eggs, consider it vegan. A vegan, after all, is not someone who's perfect. A vegan is someone who is doing his or her best to make the world a better place. A vegan could be you!

SWAP THAT SHIT

Day to day, your quest to eat vegan merely entails finding the plant-based versions of the foods you currently enjoy. Love bacon and eggs? Try scrambled tofu and tempeh bacon. Deli meat? Lightlife. Craving burgers? Duh: veggie burgers. Chicken fingers, ice cream, mac and cheese: there are vegan replacements for all of it. And we promise that you'll be surprised at how delicious it tastes. And, just like with all food, if you don't like it, just try a different brand. Virtually every food has a cruelty-free alternative, and these days all grocery stores carry vegan options. Boca, Gardein, Field Roast, Beyond Meat, and Smart Deli all make products we love. (This is not a paid brand endorsement. Yet.) Plus, since vegan staples like beans, grains, pasta, and rice are already relatively cheap, and frozen fruit and veggies keep for a long time, with a little effort, eating vegan may actually save you money. (We recommend you donate some of that dough to your favorite animal rights group.)

Even if you have a sweet tooth or consume a lot of glaucoma medication, you can still pig out. Potato chips, pretzels, Skittles, Oreos, chocolate syrup, Jolly Ranchers, Clif Bars: all vegan. That said, as our mom always reminds us: everything in moderation. Vegan junk food is still junk food. While in general a plant-based diet without dairy and hormone-injected meat can be beneficial to your health, vegans are not immune to fat. We think that just goes to show how far vegan eating has come: there are so many options that it's still possible to overeat. God bless America.

WANTS AND NEEDS

Set your long-term goal right now. What goal do you want to accomplish by the end? We normally recommend putting a date on when you want to accomplish your goal.

But one of the problems with doing that in every scenario is you start off not knowing how easy or hard it is to attain the goal.

So before you even think of a date, just simply think about the goal. Do you want to eat 100 percent vegan? Do you want to eat 90 percent vegan? Do you want to eat vegan except for weddings? Except for certain social situations?

It's totally up to you. But set your goal. For the purposes of this book we are going to make believe that everyone has the goal of eating 100 percent vegan.

Now, you can do this whatever way you want. You can commit to eat completely vegan overnight. You can do it in a week. You can do it over the next ten years.

Eating vegan is not hard. But in the beginning it is a change to get used to. But we got you. Let's do this!

Remember, don't sweat the small shit. The world we live in is amazing! But it is also kind of fucked up. It is nowhere near perfect, especially when it comes to animal cruelty and vegan eating. We need to keep things in perspective and stay focused on the long-term goals.

One way to remain focused: avoid information (the bad kind).

INFORMATION OVERLOAD

And by that, we mean shitty how-to guides.

How-to guides in the past, dictated by vegans in particular, have been known to be, well, a bit . . . what's the word? Overwhelming.

When we learn new information, and we don't have a proper way to categorize and prioritize it, the information can quickly become a disability.

It's called information overload.

You want to do this. You're ready.

But where to start?

Paralysis by analysis, as some call it, happens when someone's given you all of this info. So you've got knowledge, but you're left with no real way to effectively apply it.

This makes the knowledge next to useless. And oftentimes it can cause stress, anxiety, and sometimes depression, because you want to do it, but you feel you can't.

And it's not your fault.

"The more information the better," they say. "I give them all of the proper information. It isn't up to me to make sure they use it properly."

Oh, really? That's interesting. "Hit it and quit it" is bullshit when it comes to helping people change.

Many leaders in the past haven't learned how to help their audience achieve their goals.

They think it's just about getting the information out there. Tons of it. And then magically everyone is just going to change.

And not only that, but after they give us the

information, somehow it's our fault when they deem that we aren't taking their advice to heart.

Hey, Professor Blankity Blank, maybe you need to learn how to communicate effectively, and stop blaming shit on everyone else.

Here's an interesting thought experiment.

Do you want to summit Mount Everest today?

Of course you don't. And you can't. It's impossible.

But many how-to guides, or "leaders" (we put leaders there in quotes because many of these leaders have no real proof of success behind them) pose the move to vegan as this massive mountain you have to be determined to climb.

They frame it as though it's going to be the hardest thing you've ever done in your life. Oh, and by the way, you have to climb it all the way *today*. If you don't do it now, you're a fucking failure and I hate you.

We always ask ourselves, why the fuck are they doing that? And then we quickly realize, they just don't know any better.

They have no idea the damage they're doing to the very people they're trying to help.

> One way to motivate a switch is to shrink the change, which makes people feel 'big' relative to the challenge.
>
> —Chip and Dan Heath,
> *Switch: How to Change Things When Change is Hard*

We love that quote, and we love that book. But the sad reality is many of these guides are doing just the opposite. Rather than empowering people, they are magnifying the change into something so massive that it appears impossible, and thus becomes truly insurmountable. This creates a self-fulfilling prophecy that results in the exact opposite of what the target audience had hoped for.

There's good news. These are all methods and failings of the past. They're all correctable mistakes that well-meaning people made because they just didn't have all of the pieces to the puzzle.

They were thinking that people need to do this. But they weren't thinking, *What's the best, easiest way for anyone to do this?*

And that's really the problem here.

We're taking responsibility for that shit.

Let's leave those shortcomings and failures we just mentioned in the past. That shit is over.

With us, you're winning. There is no more losing.

And best of all, it's going to be easy. So easy, in fact, you might be like, "Why did those assholes make me think it was impossible?"

Vegan is easy as fuck. And it's only getting easier.

FUN FACT: Google saw a 90 percent increase in searches for "vegan" in 2016.

It's so easy, in fact, that there really are no "changes" required in your actual shopping or eating. It's mostly a change in mind-set. And luckily we've got you covered.

So now your eyes are open. You're ready to step into your truth. To become that superhero. To be the person you always wanted to be, but never thought you could.

And now you're likely wondering, *Where do I start?*

FAILURE IS NECESSARY

First things first.

You have our permission to . . .

FAIL.

Please fail.

Failing is important.

Why?

Failing means you're trying and working on or toward a goal.

And referencing some smart motherfuckers again, according to *New York Times* bestselling authors Dan and Chip Heath in their book *Switch*, "Failing is often the best way to learn, and because of that, early failure is a kind of necessary investment."

When sailors point their bow north, do they say, "Well, all the navigating is done because we're pointed at the North Star"? Hell no! They check their course, and when they're drifting away from north, they correct their course.

The only way for them to succeed is to notice when they're failing and correct it. Failure is key! Because the only way to fix something is to know when it's broken. Failure is simply a necessary stop on the map to success. Failure is a sign that you need a course correction.

So not only have Chip and Dan made failure acceptable for us, their research on success and change indicates that failure is necessary.

Failure is not a goal in and of itself, but it is a marker along the way. Letting us know, "Yeah bro, you've got all the right ingredients. You just added a bit of failure. Now stir a bit more and bake. You'll be there."

For many, failure is a conclusion. A sign that what you tried to do simply won't fly. You're done. Pick up the pieces and move on.

That's bullshit.

Would you quit your job if you arrived at a meeting late? Hell no! You'd note that you screwed up and resolve to do better the next time. So why is it that when people eat a slice of cheese pizza, they say, "Shit! It's all over! I can't be vegan!" Hey—you have permission to fail! Don't get discouraged!

The pressure of failure is often what causes stress, anxiety, and ultimately defeat.

We've taken all of the pressure off. You've got this and failure is a part of your new life.

And be prepared to fail more in the beginning. As we

said above, your goal isn't to fail. But it's okay. And if you fail ten years down the road, no big deal. Just look and be like, "Oh, shit. I didn't know that corn bread had eggs in it. Well, I'm glad I know now."

Fail, friends. Celebrate. And keep moving forward.

Here are some strategies to help you do exactly that.

NAME YOUR GOAL

"Jim, I've told you mine—what's your New Year's resolution this year?" Tina asked her husband as they had coffee together on January first, thinking about the year ahead.

"Oh, you know, I'd like to lose some weight at some point."

"How much and when?"

"Oh, I don't know, we'll see what happens."

You've probably heard this before. And furthermore, you've probably said this before.

Maybe you wanted to lose weight. Maybe you wanted to learn a new language, play a musical instrument, travel more, etc.

Goals are dreams with a deadline.

Dreams, on the other hand, are goals with no clear sign of completion and no deadline they must be accomplished within.

Be specific.

Jim could be clear.

"Well, Tina, I'd like to lose thirty-two pounds by December first of this year and be able to squat two hundred fifty pounds by then as well. So I can celebrate Christmas and the next new year as the person I've always wanted to be."

There's a certain magic in knowing what we want.

When we know what we want, we can naturally see more clearly how we might get there.

When we're unclear or nonspecific, we'll end up wandering through another year like Jim, never feeling moved to progress toward a goal, because we don't really know what we want.

So decide here.

When do you want to be vegetarian? When do you want to be vegan?

There is no wrong answer. You must decide on something that is equal parts doable and challenging. You should feel confident that you can accomplish it. But know that it will take work and determination to reach it.

Write it down now.

And no, you don't need to say you want to accomplish this by tomorrow. We're not trying to discourage you. But, as we've covered at length, going all in right away is typically a recipe for burnout and disaster.

Set a goal in your mind that feels right. You know what it is.

Napoleon Hill in his book *Think and Grow Rich* talks about having a definiteness of purpose.

Your goal should become a part of who you are as a person.

When we keep our goals external, they always seem like they could slip away, or be elusive and never truly attainable.

In vegan eating, this tends to happen when people don't truly believe that they are capable of being vegan.

You're in great shape. You've come this far in our book.

You agree that animal cruelty is fucked up and you want to do something about it.

You agree that the meat and dairy industries are causing catastrophic suffering to animals and the planet.

You agree that if you don't have to eat animals, well, then eating animals is kind of weird.

So you have a strong resolve.

You aren't someone tiptoeing around in "trying" to be vegan, or "trying" to eat healthier.

You know what you want, and you want it. For you. For your family. For the animals.

You want to change the world.

So think long and hard about this. Why are you doing this?

WRITE ALL OF THOSE REASONS DOWN SOMEWHERE

Wake up each day and read them. And once more, read them over before you go to sleep. This makes things more concrete, more real, more substantial. It's not just some vague wish you can't define or can't remember. It's something you've declared and committed to paper. It's real. And it's achievable.

This keeps your goal in the front of your mind. You're not putting it off. You're doing it. You're not "trying." You're becoming it!

TAKE THE EMOTION OUT

We all have ups and downs. It's life.

But when it comes to accomplishing what we want, those ups and downs can have dire consequences if we let them.

One of the big derailers of success is letting emotions take charge.

Sometimes we might not "feel" like doing it. Jim, who wants to lose thirty-two pounds by December first, is going to wake up on certain days and want to throw in the towel and eat two cakes, two pizzas, and drink a sixty-four-pack.

> **FUN FACT:** Drinking sixty-four beers in one sitting would almost surely kill you.

That's emotions laying it on thick.

But Jim has a serious case of focus. In his mind, he's already thirty-two pounds lighter. And the Jim who's thirty-two pounds lighter doesn't give in for a few minutes of junk food and skipping the gym, only to regret it all a year down the road when he's still fat.

You want to be vegan in the next three months.

You have a clear goal, and you have a definiteness of purpose.

You aren't going to let emotions dictate shit other than helping you move closer to your goal.

In your mind, you're already vegan, and someone who wants to eat vegan doesn't let emotions get them down and derail their process.

If you get down, get back up. If you fail (and you will), brush your shoulders off and move forward.

Don't let those emotions of failure spiral downward out of control and leave you feeling like nothing.

You already know you have what it takes. It's easy. You've got this.

BREAK IT DOWN

You've got your big goal: to be eating vegan in xx weeks or months.

But, let's face the truth. Weeks and months can be hard to look toward and stay optimally motivated, because well, it is quite a ways off.

It can be easy to lose focus on the finish line and get sidetracked.

That's why it's extremely important to have mini goals along the way.

Jim, who wants to lose thirty-two pounds by December first and squat 250 pounds by the same date, has a goal that is set almost an entire year in the future.

But Jim has set himself up for success in achieving his larger goal by getting there with baby steps. He breaks things down from a yearly scale to something monthly, or weekly, or daily.

One of his mini goals is to include vegetables in at least four meals a week in the beginning. He's always struggled with eating enough veggies, so he wanted to start with a realistic goal.

Once he gains confidence with the four meals per week, he'll begin upping the game, with an ultimate mini goal of consuming veggies at every meal.

In addition, he has his weekly workout goal. His weekly goal is to lift weights at the gym at least three to four times per week.

Jim has a busy schedule, and this goal allows him to make progress while also not burning himself out.

Each week he celebrates the week's victory.

Just not with a sixteen-ounce steak.

Now for his weight loss as well as his lifting goal, he breaks that shit down and celebrates the mini goals of progress along the way.

Since he wants to lose thirty-two pounds in eleven months, that takes it at about three pounds per month as an average. So he knows he wants to be losing a pound and a half at least every two weeks.

He's got his eleven-month goal, but also two-week goals to keep him highly motivated.

For squats, his plan to ultimately reach his 250-pound goal is to increase the weight at least every week. Whether it's five to ten pounds, or even just a pound or two.

You get the picture. When we break shit down into easily digestible bite-sized chunks, we begin to feel empowered along the way, rather than debilitated by a giant goal so far ahead of us.

So for you, Ms./Mr. Future Vegan of the World, we gotta make this shit easy as pie (vegan French silk pie, because it's our favorite).

You want to be vegan.

But what can you do this week?

If you feel your anxiety rising already, we need to make this small and doable.

If you're beginning this journey as a hard-core carnivore, then we begin with the classic, meatless Monday.

MEATLESS MONDAY

Yes, it's as easy as it sounds. Every Monday, you steer clear of meat. This allows you to tally wins every week, and it feels effortless.

"Hey, dude, you're not going to believe this, but I've been doing meatless Mondays for the past couple of months and it's shockingly easy."

One of Matt's best college buddies, Jefferson Hunt, a Dallas police officer, gave Matt a call one day and told him just that.

We collapsed on the floor and, once recovered, proceeded to laugh and jump for joy. Jeff was the last person either of us would ever expect to make that move. And we see shit like that every fucking day.

And he's proof how easy it is.

Jeff used to be the dude razzing Phil for being vegan. Now he's in it, moving forward and singing the praises of just how fucking easy it really is to eat more vegan food. In fact, Jeff's been feeling so confident he started leveling up. About 30–50 percent of his meals in any given week now are vegetarian or vegan.

"Okay, no offense, guys, but that is just too easy. I need more of a challenge."

Done.

Two options.

1. You could go meatless three to four days per week to start.
2. You could decide to go meatless at lunch or dinner every night.

Pick one.

Now here's where it gets more interesting. We want you to begin by simply eliminating meat at those meals.

Once you feel confident doing this, pick one or two meals each week and start exploring foods you could have in place of that meat.

We subscribe to looking at meat as a primary protein source, so in that regard we recommend exploring vegan primary protein sources.

There's a big reason for doing it this way.

People who tend to fail at the transition feel far too much pressure from the get-go to get it all right.

There's time. And we're shooting for your success to be for the rest of your life, so we're going to do this shit right.

Trying different vegan "meats" and proteins with only a meal or two each week allows you to naturally grow into your new way of life.

It will feel effortless and easy, and you can simply explore different options.

When you find something you like, make note of that, and when you find something you dislike, well, you know not to go that route anymore.

With your commitment to follow through, you are sure to find so many different foods that you enjoy, often even more than before.

There is a key when going into "trying new foods."

The right mind-set is a major key. (Shout-out to DJ Khaled.)

CHANGE YOUR MIND, CHANGE YOUR LIFE

Many who try to "change" something about their routine, their diet, their life, do not succeed because of one very important issue.

Mind-set.

We've already talked about taking the emotion out and making vegan eating a part of your identity.

Mind-set is going to be the overarching guide for this entire process, and it cannot be overstated. This is the most important part.

Those who don't succeed, don't believe. They tend to view themselves as "trying" or seeing what happens.

There's a scene in *The Karate Kid* when Mr. Miyagi asks Daniel if he's ready to begin, and Daniel, the slacker prick, says, "I guess so." Mr. Miyagi then tells him a parable of how if one walks on the right side of the road, he is safe, or the left side of the road, he is safe, but to walk down the middle, he will get squashed like a grape. You have to commit yourself to your choices. There is karate "yes" or "no," but no karate "I guess so."

And similarly in *The Empire Strikes Back* (very similarly, because Mr. Miyagi is basically Yoda and Daniel is basically Luke Skywalker, and the Cobra Kais are black-clad stormtroopers), Yoda counsels Luke, "Do. Or do not. There is no try."

FUN FACT: We think the dark side probably eats meat.

Those who succeed believe they are destined for success, which gives them a positive mental attitude going into each and every day of the journey.

The change is your Everest, and you're going to make this thing your bitch.

Let's be honest, we've gone over at length just how easy it is to eat vegan. And how it's getting easier and easier every day, week, month, and year.

Now, you wouldn't want to be one of the few losers who says, "Awww, it's too hard."

You wouldn't be able to look at yourself in the mirror, and we sure as shit wouldn't be able to look at you.

But you're an A player. You've made a decision. And you're not going back.

Failure is a part of your journey. It will only make you stronger. When you fail, you will get back up, learn your lesson, and move forward.

Vegan eating is a part of you. You've made the commitment to yourself, your family, and the animals because you're an amazing person.

Every day we want you to remind yourself how awesome you are for venturing down this path of greatness. You are becoming the superhero you never thought you could be.

Every step is a step toward changing the world, and all you have to do is simply shift what you eat a little bit.

You are the man. You are the woman. This is you now. There is no going back. Only forward.

Start each day with the positive reaffirmation that you are committed to being a badass, and it will be true.

And we'll toast to you.

DECISION WITHOUT ACTION IS BULLSHIT

If we claim success before we act, we trick our brains into giving us a dopamine drip before we actually deserve it, as though we've already accomplished our task. And this leaves us feeling good before we really should.

With Jim's weight-loss goal, if he were to just publicly go all out and tell every possible person he could that he had this goal to lose thirty-two pounds and go on and on about it, statistically he'd be very likely to fail.

When we let the cat out of the bag before we have made any actual steps in the right direction, the statistics indicate that we're most likely to not succeed at that goal.

Basically, what we're saying is keep shit quiet for a bit, and prove to yourself that you are who you say you are. Make your decision. Commit to that. Write it down.

Make it real and permanent. But you don't need to tell everyone your goal right off the bat, or you're going to feel too much pressure. First decide, but back up that decision with action, not just words.

For years you've stated that you're against animal cruelty. Don't talk about it. Be about it. But start small and then build up.

The first and only real person the decision matters to right now is you.

As you gain confidence and come into your own, you're proving to yourself that you are that person.

Now that your actions are lining up and your resolve to stick with it is bulletproof, you can start letting people know.

At this point you'll be solidifying your new way of life with each person close to you that finds out.

Because now our brain wants us to stay consistent with who we say we are. So letting Mom and Dad know at this point, even if it's a sticky subject for them, will actually benefit you. Because you are telling yourself, "I am who I say that I am, and you will not deter me."

You will begin to feel more powerful in every aspect of your life.

Being a person of your word.

Feeling incredible for doing your part.

Feeling confident for accomplishing a goal you set out.

Feeling happy because you are in alignment with who you truly want to be.

Feeling more attractive and magnetic because you are living your truth now for the world to see, and you're a genuinely more upbeat, happy, and positive person.

Call it karma. Call it the power of doing good. Call it supernatural. Call it whatever the fuck you want.

But trust us when we say, life gets amazing from this point on.

PRACTICAL GUIDE

People feel overwhelmed. "Oh, but what are you going to eat?" "Where will you get your protein?"

These are the lies the meat and dairy industries have been whispering in our ears for years.

Thank God their lies are over, and you're seeing the light.

Gone are the days of difficulty.

The future is here now, though. And it's easier and tastier than ever.

Now that we've told you some of our strategies and techniques for achieving your vegan dreams, let's look at a very detailed battle plan that we've found to be highly effective. This will give a step-by-step, week-by-week course of action for how to get on the vegan train. Come with us on the journey.

THE VEGAN BROS RECOMMENDED PLAN

The next time you hit the grocery store, you're going to mostly view it as a normal grocery shopping trip. You're going to buy all the same shit you normally buy, but you're also going to try some new shit as well. So get ready to throw some new stuff into your cart.

> **FUN FACT:** Whole Foods is our favorite grocery store in the entire world. Our second favorite grocery store is the Amazon Fresh page at amazon.com. But vegan eating is easy at almost every grocery store.

Weeks One to Three

Your goal for this week and the next week is to just try some of the various plant-based options. Discover the options you don't like, the options you do like, experiment with cooking them, etc. Obviously, you'll be exploring new food for the rest of your life. But exploring is the only goal for the first three weeks.

Remember, this is just our *recommended* plan. If you need a longer time, that's fine. Just keep the long-term goal in your head.

Don't just buy one or two products on this shopping trip.

Think about all the products with meat in them that you don't like, like gefilte fish and SPAM. Now imagine if you had just tried those two items and decided you hated meat.

It's the same thing for food without meat. Just because you think one vegan product is the shittiest thing you've ever eaten, it doesn't mean the fifty thousand other products are shit, too. Everyone has the food they hate and the food they love. So make sure you leave yourself room to not like something but still like some other shit.

You're going to head to the frozen aisle. It could be the regular frozen aisle. But it could also be in some sort of natural food aisle as well. Different grocery stores put this shit in different areas.

You're going to look for brands like Boca, Field Roast, Gardein, and Beyond Meat. You'll see different products from these brands like chicken nuggets, brats, beefless tips, burgers, etc. You also may find Daiya pizzas, Amy's burritos, and other amazing shit. Load that shit in your cart. As much as you want.

If you haven't been one to explore eating much fruit or vegetables, feel free to do that shit as well. It's all about exploring right now. Try a pineapple. Experiment with some baby bok choy and garlic—it's fucking delicious.

Continue shopping this way for about three weeks.

And during these first three weeks you're going to choose one of these two options:

- Commit to eating vegan at least one full day per week.
- Commit to eating a vegan breakfast, a vegan lunch, and a vegan dinner on different days.

Doing this allows you to not feel overwhelmed by the change. It allows you to approach it at a speed that feels comfortable to you. One full day of eating vegan? That's one out of seven. And three meals for the rest of the week? That's three out of the remaining eighteen. That's not too much. If you scored a 3/18 on a test, you'd fail in any college in the country. But with our plan? That's a win, bro!

Weeks Four and Five

After you get a bit of a grasp on the food, at about the fourth week you're going to buy slightly less of the meat and dairy products you used to buy. You don't need to eliminate them completely just yet, unless you feel comfortable doing so.

And if there is still one product in particular you can't view yourself giving up, don't give it up yet. For example, if you have ever said something like, "I would go vegan, but I could never give up cheese (or insert any other animal product)," don't give it up yet. You're thinking long term right now. So don't feel the need to go all in just yet.

Think about the new vegan foods you liked that you bought in the previous three weeks. Load up on that shit this week.

Now think about one meat product you normally buy, but enjoy eating the least. Buy a little less of that this week, or maybe just don't buy it at all. View it as replacing that animal product with the new vegan products you like.

You want the goal to be doable. But you also want the goal to take you out of your comfort zone.

The goal for the next two weeks is to add another day of vegan eating to your life. At this point, do two full days of vegan eating if you feel it's possible.

Weeks Six to Fourteen

You're going to repeat this process every two weeks. This means that by week fourteen, you will be eating vegan 100 percent of the time or very close to it.

Remember, don't feel the need to be rigid with this shit. We obviously encourage you to eat vegan every single time you eat. But you make the rules. And you can make any exceptions you want.

If you eat 100 percent vegan for nine months, but then eat meat at one social function, that's fine. Just keep doing what you're doing. Pretty soon that social function will be vegan anyway. But we need you to stay on board even if you relapse once in a while. (Side note: Your body might not react so well to eating meat once every nine months. Fair warning.)

There's how-to guides for transitioning to a vegan diet all over the place. They're a dime a dozen nowadays.

But there are some flaws in the process, and we're going to fix them for you.

Learn from this common how-to guide mistake.

MEAL PLANS

Most guides give meal plans that they encourage participants to follow.

It looks right. It sounds right. And it works for some people.

But it's not quite right for the majority of people.

There's no flexibility for the real life you live. And there's no real transfer of knowledge and power to you as an individual.

When people are simply told to follow meal plans, they can feel good in the beginning. Like, "Oh man, I can do this."

Just buy this, this, and this and we're good.

Blind obedience can be liberating. Nothing to have to think about!

But what happens when you start to get sick of the meal plans? The meal plans are the foundation for the way those folks are eating. And so if you can't do them, you can't stick to your new path.

A few months, or a year down the road, people drop out. They don't really know how the meal plans are made up, or why they should be doing things a certain way.

People end up ultimately feeling disempowered and uneducated. Rather than large feelings of having an impact on the world, you're stuck looking at the fucking meal plan every fucking day. Fuck. That. Shit.

Most people don't want to feel like they need to learn an entire new system, or a new way of life. And they also don't want to feel like they're stuck in the same place just listening to someone dictate to them in the kitchen for the rest of their life.

In addition to the lack of education, people just generally end up feeling boxed in. And we all know what happens to people who feel boxed in. Eventually, it implodes in some way.

You want this. You want to take full ownership; you want this to be a permanent and effortless part of your life. You want this to be part of your lifestyle that you fully understand, can easily explain, and can work with on the fly. Whether you're at home with the family, traveling, or, fuck, even in the middle of nowhere needing a quick bite.

Meal plans won't get you there.

And ultimately will result in high recidivism.

Blindly jump in face-first and step into the scary unknown.

That sounds doable, doesn't it?

When Sergey Brin and Larry Page started Google, they had a simple but very understandable goal they spelled out: don't be evil.

Does it seem too simple? Maybe. But those guys seem to know a thing or two about success. And their plan is fairly similar to our plan: state your goal and write it down. Don't get bogged down in too much minutiae. Keep it simple. Our vegan plan might be titled something similar, like "Don't Be an Asshole."

How can you achieve your goal of being a vegan and not being an asshole? Don't be an ingredient nazi. Start small and build up from there. Don't try to be perfect. Don't be afraid to fail. Don't sweat the small shit. Name your goal. Articulate your reasons for making a change. Remind yourself of those reasons often. Take the emotion out of it. Break shit down into doable chunks. Get your mind-set right. Make bold decisions but marry them with actions.

And have fun.

Going vegan isn't a hardship—it's a liberation! There's a whole new world of food out there for you to discover, and it's going to be a blast sampling it all! It's a change, and it's a change that's going to take some adjustment, but it's also a change that you're going to discover you love.

It's a big world out there. Take a bite!

CHAPTER 8

YOU WANT TO TAKE THIS SHIT OUTSIDE?: VEGAN ON THE ROAD

EVER GO TO A PARTY at a friend's new house? Or a new friend's house? It can be a different experience. If you've got friends who entertain a lot, you know that going to their house is going to be awesome—it's going to have food, it's going to have drinks, there are going to be lots of interesting people there—you can book that as a win. But when it's a new friend or a new place? Then you don't know the layout of the place, you don't know if you have to take your shoes off when you get in . . . but it's still going to be awesome! Because parties are fun! And even if they're unfamiliar, then they're still going to have food and drinks and interesting people, because . . . it's a *party*!

And eating vegan outside the home can be like going to a party in a place you've never been to before. Sure, there are going to be some things you didn't plan on (there's a bathtub in the living room? Okay. Caprese salad skewers are a thing? Fine, I'll chomp on that shit), but it's still going to be a blast, and you're going to have a great time.

In the last chapter, we talked about how to develop a game plan to switch to vegan eating at home. Now we're going to look at some tools and techniques that will make it super easy and super fun to eat vegan on the road.

When you're at home, you control all the ingredients and get to make all the decisions. So you've got a lot of power. But even when you're going outside, you still have a ton of power. Remember—you're not going to be taking a rocket to Mars. You're just going to a party! Eating vegan out is a snap—but it never hurts to have a few strategies and techniques to make it even easier.

You got this.

RESTAURANTS (PLACES YOU EAT FOOD)

Don't think for a second you need to prepare all your meals at home with garden-grown ingredients and recyclable silverware. You are not a dirty hippie. (Maybe you're a clean one.) We want you to go out to eat just like you normally would. But at the same time, you have to understand that there are a few different rules to eating in your home versus eating in a restaurant. For instance, you have to wear pants. And you'll probably be expected to use some kind of utensil(s). It's a buzzkill, sure, but that's the reality. So far, so good. We know that this is all pretty earth-shattering, but we can get you through these trying times.

Here are a couple of other things for an enterprising young vegan *not* to do upon entering a restaurant:

1) Ask: "Is the beer vegan?"
2) Ask: "Is the bread vegan?"
3) Ask: "Are the vegetables cooked on the same grill as the meat?"
4) Leave without ordering.

Eating vegan at restaurants is easy shit. But you'd be surprised by how often we hear stories and comments like you see above. Even though some vegans have good intentions, they lose sight of what's important. Veteran vegan advocate Bruce Friedrich says: "Your pursuit of personal purity in that instance does significantly more harm to animals than consuming that tiny bit of animal product." This is a handy reminder: it's not about you. It's about the animals. Let's not forget why most animals are being killed, tortured, and abused: the consumption of meat, fish, dairy, and eggs. If the vegetables are cooked on the same grill as the meat, there's nothing (within reason) you can do about it. And that's okay.

And have you ever seen a restaurant kitchen? It's cramped. It's chaotic. It's hot as shit and full of stress and adrenaline. It's NOT the kind of place where the owner says, "Shit—I've got tons of extra room! Let's have one grill just for red meat, one for chicken, one for fish, one for vegetables, and some special buffer grills separating all of them, each MADE OF SOLID GOLD!" Hell no! That shit would be hard to find. So when you ask things like "Can my vegetables be grilled on a different appliance than the meat" to the server and everyone at your table, it sounds like you're saying, "Can my food be made separate from all the other food, just for me, because I'm such a fucking special snowflake?" Sure, your intentions may be right, but good job, you just made everyone at your table think eating vegan is hard. And if you've ever been guilty of this in the past, just apologize and promise never to do it again. No big deal!

And is the bread vegan? Eventually, all bread will be made without dairy. And right now, most of the time there isn't any dairy. But sometimes the bread will have some sort of dairy product in it. It's best for your friends to not hear you ask a question like, "Is there any dairy in the bread?" If they don't hear you ask that, they'll be a million times more likely to consider eating vegan in the future. Also, you want to have a positive impact on the server.

When vegans give servers at restaurants the third degree about their menu, they're turning off not only the server, but also the kitchen staff, and even fellow diners. Now all those people are *less* likely to eat vegan because you were more concerned with personal purity than the animals we're trying to save.

We do realize, though, that some of you are new to this, and eating out can throw a few curveballs every now and then. So we have a few tried-and-true tips to help you succeed.

TIPS FOR SUCCESS ON THE OUTSIDE

- Know before you go: happycow.net and vegguide.org are both great resources for finding vegan-friendly restaurants.
- Do your best. It's okay if you're not 10,000 percent certain that your meal is 100 percent vegan—though we appreciate your enthusiasm!
- It's okay to ask your server a few questions. Just don't grill him or her like she's under oath for Benghazi. Remember, you are representing the motherfucking animals!
- If all else fails, order the veggie burger. Even the most podunk, backwoods rib joints have veggie burgers

these days. One hack we love for health reasons is to request (nicely) that the veggie burger be cut up over a salad. Done.

- Get creative. On the rare occasion where there is absolutely nothing truly vegan on the entrée menu, you can oftentimes combine a few different smaller options, like steamed vegetables or beans or avocado, into one great vegan meal.

- Treat the waitstaff with respect, tip a little extra, and make sure you review the restaurant on Yelp to let everyone know how well they accommodated you. Give credit where credit is due!

LAND(S) OF PLENTY

We've found that even the major chains are looking out for vegans and vegetarians these days. Taco Bell—yes, *Taco Bell*—has a vegetarian menu certified by the American Vegetarian Association. That is probably our favorite vice while hammered or hungover, or while having hunger pangs on a long road trip. Buffalo Wild Wings has a great black bean burger. We like to eat it on a bun or over their garden salad (hold the cheese). Red Robin has a killer veggie burger that we enjoy with their unlimited steak fries. Even Subway has vegetable patties you can get as a sub or on a salad. Eat fresh, indeed.

Perhaps the most variety and flavor you can get while

eating vegan is by trying ethnic food. We've traveled the world (with our taste buds, at least) to find the most delicious vegan fare from any ethnicity.

- Mexican: Bean burrito with rice and veggies and a side of chips (ask for no cheese or sour cream). Sometimes there is lard in the beans, and chicken stock in the rice. Feel free to politely ask if you want. But it's up to you.
- Chinese: Vegetable spring rolls for an appetizer. Any rice or noodle dish with vegetables and tofu for your entrée. And pick whatever sauces you want! (Sometimes egg noodles and fish sauce are used at Chinese restaurants. Feel free to ask.)
- Indian: Phil loves vegetable samosas, and there are tons of vegetable-based entrees to try, but a word of warning: Indian food will often include yogurt or cream in the sauces. Just make sure to ask your server politely when you order.
- Middle Eastern: Deep-fried falafel sandwich with veggies and tahini sauce. You can also eat pitas and hummus to your heart's content.
- Japanese: We both love avocado rolls, but obviously any vegetable sushi will do.
- Italian: Pasta with marinara sauce, motherfucker.

One of the nice things about eating in ethnic restaurants is that they often base their menus on places that don't get

TONS of meat. So these regions have spent hundreds or thousands of years devising ways to make vegetables delicious. Try some *mesir wat* (lentil stew) at an Ethiopian restaurant or vegetable *panang* curry at a Thai place (ask for no fish sauce just in case), or some vegetable pho at a Vietnamese restaurant. Pho is Matt's single favorite meal in the history of the world. If you want to do it like him, be sure to douse it with Sriracha. You will not be disappointed!

> **FUN FACT:** Pho is delicious. And Bamboo on 15th Avenue in Capitol Hill, Seattle, makes some of the best vegan pho in the entire world.

Did you get a little hungry reading this? 'Cause we got a little hungry writing it. But it just proves how many awesome delicious vegan options there are for dining out. If you're hesitant about eating vegan while out, one thing you don't have to worry about is not being able to hang with your friends or order on dates. Eating vegan is a cinch and, at the end of the day, we're a lot less annoying than those gluten-free motherfuckers.

PARTIES

Okay, so there are tons of ways to make trips to restaurants more inviting. That's easy. But what happens if you get invited to someone's home, for a dinner party or some other party? What do you do then?! Spoiler alert: it's also easy.

First, don't panic. There's no need to worry, for a bunch of reasons. For one thing, the entire world is going to be eating vegan pretty quickly, so you're going to be encountering lots of people sympathetic to your needs. The odds of you encountering a situation where you're going to feel on the outs is pretty slim. And in the rare instance you do encounter someone like that, you may as well feel sorry for that person, because everyone hates them. You just need to follow a few simple rules about eating out.

The first rule of eating vegan is never leaving the house. So problem solved. The end!

No, no, no. It's actually important that you venture out into the world if you're vegan. (Cue theme song from Disney's *Aladdin*—"A Whole New World") And the problems you may encounter aren't going to be big steeplechase obstacles, they're just tiny little inconveniences. The kind of obstacles you might encounter on a speed-walk course. You know, a few leaves and the occasional bumbling ant. Obstacles that don't require Olympic-level athleticism to negotiate. And if you're going to a vegan's house for a party, that's probably pretty safe, too.

You know what else is safe?

Everyone's house.

It's true. Even if you've got some truly clueless friends who don't know that you eat vegan, or know that you're vegan but don't know what that means, or know what it means but don't give a shit, it's still pretty safe to go to pretty much anyone's house for a party. Even if there's literally nothing for you to eat, just bacon served on pork chops, the smell of cooking meat won't make you pass out from meat fumes. So in a worst-case scenario, you come, you hang out, you drink a few beers, and you go get some Taco Bell on the way home. You came. You partied. You showed everyone you're a winner. And you left. Not exactly a disaster. And that's probably the very worst case we can think of.

Well, the *very* worst case would be if you went to this party, and some very aggressive meat-eating guests held you down and force-fed you burgers that have mad cow disease. But that occurs *very* rarely, and really is probably the worst-case scenario.

That being said, even the noncrazy worst-case scenario isn't exactly the end of the world. Some people are less thoughtful than others, but it's really not a big deal.

DOS AND DON'TS

Do: Bring something. This is actually just good advice on being a fucking adult. If someone invites you to a party (a Super Bowl party, an Oscar party, a dinner party, it applies to them all), it's polite to bring a bottle of wine, a six-pack of beer, a baguette, a bottle of vodka. No? Okay, maybe that's just us, but bring *something*.

Don't just show up empty-handed! And if you're a vegan, you can show up with some spring rolls or some crudité (chopped mixed vegetables, you unsophisticated slobs!) or some chips and dip. Then, if there's nothing else to eat, you can just eat what you brought.

Don't: Tell your host that you're a vegan and that they should include some vegan options, or risk being labeled an asshole. That's kind of a shitty move. We had a friend who would call up his friends when they announced a party and say things like, "I've been eating Italian all week, so don't serve any pasta on Saturday," or, "I'm in the mood for something spicy, so would it kill you to have some nachos or something?" Would the hosts feel guilted or shamed into catering to this guy's whims? Yeah. Did he get what he wanted at least half the time? Amazingly, yes. Did he get invited to a lot of parties after pulling that shit? No, he didn't. You're going to a party, not a restaurant, so don't treat the hosts like they're the help (also, don't forget what we said about restaurants).

Do: Eat ahead of time. This is somewhat party-specific. If you're going to a party of sixty-year-olds, there's a good chance they won't have a lot of vegan options, because older people can be a little behind the times, unless they're our parents. Then they're vegan. But square television sets. Dial-up Internet. The use of travel agents.

And it would be a bummer to show up at a party expecting to chow down on food to find that it's just cheese and crackers and salami. If that's the kind of soiree you're expecting, just eat what you want beforehand, and then have a few beers or glasses of wine at the party. If it's something like a dinner party, you can't quite pull that move, because then you're showing up full to a party where the whole point is to feed you, and that's sort of showing a big middle finger to your hosts, saying, "I figured you'd fucking suck at feeding me, so I did it myself."

Again, it depends a bit on who's running the show. If it's nice people, then they'll probably have something for you and you can throw caution to the wind. If they're a little behind the times, you might want to have a little something before you go out, and then just plan on eating side dishes. Brussels sprouts and salad for dinner. No big deal. And if it's forty-year-olds in Brooklyn, we think there's a law that all the food has to be vegan anyway, so you're golden.

Don't: Be a preachy asshole. Phil learned this lesson when we were younger and he insulted a guest at a party for wearing fur. Did he make his point by calling her a murderer? Yes. Did he convince everyone else at the party that fur was a bad thing? No, he did not, though he did convince everyone else at the party that antifur crusaders were a bunch of preachy assholes who need a good beating. Similarly, you shouldn't go to a party hoping to convert people by insulting them. "You're eating meat? You realize that you're going to hell, don't you?" That's a party foul. Lead by example, gracefully and with good humor. If someone asks if you're vegan, respond honestly. If they ask why you're a vegan, feel free to tell them. But don't corner someone against the bookshelf and tell them how you received the Medal of Seitan from Miley Cyrus (we love you, Miley) back in '15 and that eating chicken wings is murder, because that just makes all vegans look like crazy narcissists. Parties are for people to have a good time, not for passionate vegans to prey upon a captive audience.

We once went to a party where the host, who was learning guitar, decided to break it out and sing songs for her guests for OVER AN HOUR! Why didn't people leave? Partly, it was because everyone thought the last song would be the final song, but mostly it was because people are polite. They listened to her songs because they felt an obligation to, but they weren't having a good time. And people might listen to you harangue them for twenty minutes out of pure human decency, but that doesn't mean you're convincing them of anything other than the fact that you're an overaggressive prick.

Do: Be adventurous. By this, I don't mean that you should eat a plate of baby back ribs if offered to you, but you should always be thinking of fun ways to expand your choices, rather than narrow them (and this applies to meat eaters as well!). So if you're at a party and the only nonmeat entrée is borscht, and you've never had it before, don't say, "Beets are for peasants—begone with ye!" Instead, give it a try. You might like it, and even if you don't, you're a fucking adult—prove it! If a host offers some food that you're unfamiliar with, and it's vegan-approved, give it a whirl. It would be bad form to show up at a dinner party and push away the rice noodles, the orzo and pine nut salad, and the coconut curry soup and say, "I mostly eat veggie burgers." Someone makes an effort to make you happy, you have to meet them halfway and at least try it. Don't force yourself to choke down a meal you don't like, but live a little!

Don't: Lie. For a lot of vegans, avoiding meat and meat products is a choice, not a necessity. We can literally digest meat, but just choose not to (for some pretty fucking justifiable reasons). This might mean that hosts at parties might think it's not a necessity to cater to our diets. And them's the breaks and life goes on. But that doesn't mean that people should try to influence the menu at a party by lying. We once had a friend who went to an Irish pub that served burgers on poppy seed buns, and she didn't like the idea of poppy seeds getting stuck in her teeth and making her look gross in photos, so she told the waiter that she was deathly allergic to them, and to remove the seeds but still serve the buns. Poppy seeds are small as shit, so the waiter said he couldn't guarantee that he'd be able to extract every one of the 6 million poppy seeds from the bun, and could she perhaps eat the burger without the bun? She replied that she'd prefer the bun, and that she was just making up the allergy because she thought he'd be more likely to accommodate her weird request. He said, "I'm not serving you food you said would kill you two minutes ago." And even if you think that it might tip the scales in your favor of getting food you want, don't tell hosts at a party some shit like, "I've got a heart condition, and any meat in the room could give me a fucking coronary," or, "I have a sensitivity to fish, and ingesting any will cause my dick to fall off." Sure, that's going to make people take your dietary needs ultra-seriously, but you're basically hijacking a party that way. Stick to the truth—it's easier to remember. And we're going to win this thing anyway, so let's not taint our legacy with any vegan Ballgazis or Deflategates.

DATING

How does being vegan affect the dating scene? Does being vegan make it harder to date?

Not really. Dating while vegan is pretty simple these days. There are lots of options out there. It's sort of like picking a paint for your house (assuming you own the house—if you paint your building and you're just renting one unit, painting it might actually cause some problems). Yeah, you'll look through a few samples first, but you'll find something you like.

For dating advice, we turn to the timeless wisdom of Sun Tzu's *The Art of War*. Now, we're not trying to make a statement that dating is a war, and that one can only be victorious if one defeats his or her dating partner, but bear with us. Sun Tzu addresses many aspects of warfare, including the use of spies, terrain, deceit, and tactics. One of the most famous lines from his masterwork is "Every battle is won or lost before it is fought." In other words, the preparation for an engagement will decide the engagement. So plan accordingly!

And this can apply to anything. Anticipating the first day of class? Then bring some paper and something to write with. Not a big deal. Moving to a new apartment? Make sure to get plenty of boxes and packing tape before the big move. Again, not rocket science. This shit kind of takes care of itself. You don't need to bring peace to the Middle East or anything. We're talking about making a pretty simple thing even easier, so you can chill out.

If you're vegan, and you're asking someone to a dinner date, do a little reconnaissance first. You want to make sure that the place you go has options for everyone. So don't just suggest, "We should get some dinner. I hear that place on the corner is super packed every night." No, no, no! Don't just pick a place because it's trendy! You've already lost the battle! Maybe it's trendy because it has a celebrity chef who will charge you $100 a plate for croutons. Maybe it's trendy because it employs some idiotic gimmick to get people in the door, like having people eat on beds or on the floor (two different *Sex and the City* plotlines, amazingly). And do you want to go to some place that's packed for dinner? Absolutely not! You might have to wait hours to get in, or you might only be able to eat if you show up super early or super late. And—and this is the most important detail—THEY MIGHT NOT SERVE FOOD YOU LIKE! It seems obvious that one should go to restaurants that they know serves food they would want to eat, but not everyone seems to understand this. So if you're vegan, don't just suggest a place because your friend who loves steaks recommended it. Do a little research, verify that the menu would agree with you, and then suggest it.

Now, this is not to say that you should always pick strictly vegan restaurants! If you're vegan, and you're trying to select a nice place for dinner, DON'T choose a vegan restaurant. Why? Because maybe your date isn't vegan (yet)! While we think the world would be a better place if everyone were vegan, we don't think that it's going to convince people to go vegan by being too aggressive. If you want to convince a nonvegan that eating vegan is the way to go, you will be far more convincing by leading by example, by showing that you can satisfy all your needs with the choices already out there. Vegan restaurants are fantastic, but one of the great things about eating vegan is that you don't have to eat at only vegan eateries in order to eat vegan! That's kind of a tongue twister, but it's still true!

If you take someone out to dinner at a nonvegan restaurant, then you can show that you can find delicious choices even when your specific dietary needs aren't being catered to. "Check me out! I'm at Taco Bell, and I'm still eating vegan and loving it!" Though we don't suggest you take a date to Taco Bell. Go to a place that has waiters that come to the table and where the utensils are made of metal. Because classy.

This is not to say that you can't go to a vegan restaurant somewhere down the line, but on a first date, you're trying to get to know someone, not trying to convert someone. Insisting on eating at a vegan restaurant on a first date might come off as uncompromising, so just go to a nice Italian restaurant and see how it goes!

What about if you're vegan and you're the one being asked out—does that change your options at all? It does alter things a little bit, since you have to be more reactive than active, but *The Art of War* still applies. If someone asks you out, and you want to go out with them, say yes, then find out where they're thinking of taking you. Don't lead off with a list of restaurants that you want, because that might come off as pretty demanding.

Just say, "Thanks for the invite! I'd love to have dinner

with you!" Then, later, when they're talking about the details, the vegan who is being asked out can just investigate the menu at their leisure. If they see that there aren't enough nonmeat options, they can just call or text or e-mail or singing telegram the asker and say, "I was just looking at the menu and I realized that I'm really craving either pasta or Thai. What do you think about that?"

No fuss, no muss, no ultimatums. You don't have to say, "I'm vegan and must go to vegan-approved eateries." That can be a tough prerequisite, and it also gives other vegans a bad reputation as being pushy and uncompromising.

In both cases, a little preparation can be a good thing. It sounds simple and helpful, but not everyone inherently understands this. We had a friend, Terrance, who was lazy as shit. Just didn't put in a lot of effort. When he would ask someone out, he would focus mostly on geography. He'd want to ask out someone who lived in his neighborhood, so he wouldn't have to travel very far to see her in case things worked out, and he'd want to eat at someplace in his neighborhood, so he wouldn't have to travel very far for the date. Already, that's pretty damn lazy. But there's more! He wouldn't just say, "Hey, baby, let's go to this French place at the end of my block so I don't have to cross the street and risk putting a crease in my new kicks." He would be so lazy, he'd just suggest shit like, "Hey, let's meet up near my apartment and just walk a block or two to find something that looks good."

Can you believe that shit? This was a battle LOST before it was ever fought, because Terrance was too lazy to do the barest amount of work ahead of time. His dates would always find it weird, and would also instantly think Terrance was just this flaky dude who couldn't express a preference for a restaurant. Now, to be fair to him, he was doing this in part because he didn't want to just act unilaterally and pick a place his date might not like, but that's why people do research! And talk! Do a little prep work ahead of time, and everyone will benefit.

Eating out can be a lot of fun. But it can also create some challenges. Unfamiliarity can be stressful. New settings can be awkward. But they can also be exciting and stimulating, and there are tools and strategies you can use to ensure you have a great time eating out.

We both ate meat for a long time. There's nothing we can do about the animals that suffered in the past as a result. But we can work to change it in the future. Still, there will be times when the restaurant screws up, or a product is mislabeled, or, hell, you just accidentally stick something in your mouth without thinking. It's okay. You got this. You're doing something amazing. Be proud of making the world a better place.

And when someone looks at you and says, "Holy shit! You're the greatest person in the world. What should I do?"

Just look at them and say, "Join me. We're taking over."

CHAPTER 9

FOLLOW THE BILLIONS: THE FUTURE OF FOOD

So NOW YOU KNOW how to make the transition to eating vegan, both behind closed doors and right in the middle of Main Street. But the world changes quickly. What does the future hold for meatless eating?

We're sure the future will have lots of pretty cool things. Like flying cars, and computer chips that you can install in your brain to record both every visual image and every bit of trivia, and clothes that are all shiny and formfitting to make people look like foiled-up baked potatoes (which are also vegan), and hackers that break into the server that operates robotic bees and programs them to burrow into your brain and make you scream in agony (sorry, we've been watching too much *Black Mirror* on Netflix lately).

For the most part, the future sounds pretty amazing. But there will also be some significant challenges. Every day, the world makes more people, and every day, those people have fewer and fewer resources to share. The UN predicts that by 2050, Earth's population will soar to almost 10 billion people. So . . . what are all those people going to eat?!

One way to get a preview of what the future might bring is to see where the venture capitalists, the top companies, and the R&D people put their money. Money is always a reliable indicator. Ever see *All the President's Men*? Great movie. When Woodward is talking to Deep Throat, he's told that he'll make progress if he were to "follow the money." There are lots of smart people out there, and they sometimes manage to acquire shitloads of money. Where they put their money is often proof of where things are headed. Just got to follow the money. And also the flavor.

Now obviously there are innovations happening all over food. From vertical farming vegetables to harvesting algae to 3-D printing of food to eating meals in pill form, there's a lot of crazy shit going on out there. But the most important innovations in food are in meat, or more to the point, replicating and/or replacing it. Or, more basically, keeping the meat, but removing the animal.

Capitalism is vegan, people. The money is flowing in, and it's not going toward new ways of shredding chickens and cows.

MEAT (FROM PLANTS)

What can about $100 million in VC funding from investors like Google and Bill Gates get you in Silicon Valley? The next Facebook? The next Uber? Well, it might just buy you the next hamburger. Specifically, the perfect plant-based burger, courtesy of California start-up Impossible Foods and their secret ingredient: heme.

What is heme? It sounds like the adorable comic relief animal sidekick in a Disney animated movie ("Thanks for the help, Heme the platypus!"), but heme is the secret ingredient to a seriously delicious burger—and a burger made from 0 percent cow! The burger is made from wheat, coconut oil, and potatoes. And heme. Heme is an iron-containing, oxygen-carrying compound that makes meat smell, sizzle, bleed, and taste amazing (the heme in cows is in the form of hemoglobin). Heme occurs in about ten parts per million in beef, and about two parts per million in chicken. But if you add some heme to chicken, it starts tasting like beef. So what if one could take that awesome magic compound and somehow add it to a burger made from plants? You get a burger that smells, tastes, and sizzles like meat!

The brainchild of Stanford chemistry professor Patrick W. Brown, Impossible Foods uses cutting-edge technology to identify what makes food delicious and engineers that into their all-plant burger. They use a straight-from-*CSI* (or

NCIS or any of the other forensic procedurals—they're all pretty much the same) gas chromatograph mass spectrometer (CG-MS) to analyze the flavors and smells produced when grilling both traditional meat and plant-based meat in order to create a noncow burger that is virtually indistinguishable from a classic beef burger. Except, you know, less ripping out of throats and fewer eviscerations.

It wasn't easy to engineer the burger. Just finding a good, representative sample of what they wanted to emulate proved a bit of a challenge. Why? Because after sampling three hundred different kinds of ground beef, from the bargain bin at a local supermarket to the rarefied air of Kobe, they ALL tested positive for shit. Literally, every single sample was contaminated at some level with feces. Cow feces, we assume, but who knows? Maybe someone in the slaughterhouse was taking a dump in the stun line. That's another nice benefit to plant-based meats: the plants don't shit themselves nearly as much as the cows (or, perhaps more accurately, the plants don't have bowels that can get perforated during slaughter that can then spread over the carcass). But the food scientists found the right sample, they did their magic, and they found their heme.

Heme isn't unique to animal flesh. Plants also have heme, and hemoglobin, and Impossible Foods found their ideal source of heme in soy root nodules. So even though heme is what gives their meat its bloody juices and flavor, they're not actually just dumping blood in their veggies. They're using the heme in veggies to make it taste just like meat! They took some soy DNA that codes for heme, and inserted it into some yeast. And the yeast then produces this plant blood! Freaky? A little. Delicious? You better believe it.

These food scientists also had to engineer the proteins necessary to give their burger the right mouthfeel, the right bounce, so that biting into a mouthful of veggies would feel just like biting into a Quarter Pounder and not chewing on a mouthful of dandelions (an important part of selling burgers, apparently). To simulate muscle tissue, they used wheat and potato proteins. To simulate connective tissues, they used soybeans and wheat gluten. And to mimic the fat of a burger? Coconut oil. The final flavor enhancer to make it taste like beef? Honeydew melon. Who would have thought?!

> **FUN FACT:** Americans are really starting to love veggie burgers.

They tinkered with the formula, dialing back on the honeydew, adjusting the levels, until they finally had a burger made entirely from veggies that tastes like a burger made entirely from cows. Could it be the future of the burger?

Lots of people think so. And it's not just vegans, either. You know who else wants in on the plant-based meat revolution? Tyson!

Tyson?! That seems wrong. After all, Tyson Foods makes $41 billion a year primarily through its sales of chicken, beef, and pork. But that didn't stop them from buying a 5 percent minority share in the California-based vegan startup Beyond Meat. Beyond Meat also received funding from Biz Stone and Evan Williams, the founders of Twitter.

Why would Tyson be interested in vegan foods? For the fucking money! According to the Plant-Based Foods Association, sales of plant-based food products rang in about almost $5 billion from June 2015 to June 2016, and grew faster than the overall food business.

General Mills also invested in Beyond Meat. Because apparently, the food giant actually wants to keep making money in the future. Crazy, right? But they can see the writing on the wall. Killing cows and chickens is on the way out, and if they want to stay in business, they're going to have to stay ahead of the trends. In the business world, where it's kill or be killed, the way to keep making a killing is to stop with all the killing, apparently.

Beyond Meat makes a ton of our favorite products, but they recently outdid themselves by producing a plant-based burger that rivals beef. One of their patties has about the same amount of protein as a regular beef burger, half the saturated fat, and no cholesterol. The protein for their burger actually comes mostly from peas. Ever watch one of those videos of heart surgery, where the doctors scrape away a bunch of gunk that's clogging a heart? Ever hear any of the doctors say something like, "Wow—look at all this pea fat"? No, we didn't think so.

This is huge! We've talked about all the ways that animal-based products can't compete with plant-based products, that they're cruel, they're ruinous to the environment, they create pollution, and so on. So there are only two ways that animal-based foods can resist the vegan revolution: taste and price. And now companies like Beyond Meat and Impossible Foods have basically closed the gap on taste! It's only a matter of time. Because when you've got taste on your side, more people are going to eat your food (because that's just fucking rocket science, right?), and the more people eat your food, the cheaper it becomes to produce. (We learned that in college 'cause we're smart) So plant-based proteins are just going to get tastier and cheaper. And you know what that means? It means consumers are going to look at a menu, or survey the options at the supermarket, and say, "Well, one option is cheaper and healthier and tastier, but the other option causes all this evil shit. That's a tough decision . . ."

We mean, who is going to go for option two in that scenario?! It's pretty much just James Bond villains and sentient potatoes who don't want to engage in cannibalism.

That's the list. When there's no incentive to eat animal protein, that's going to collapse lightning quick.

MEAT EXTENDERS!

Yeah, you hear something like "meat extenders," and you think that it sounds like a dodgy, low-budget late-night infomercial. "Having trouble in the bedroom? Well, kiss those troubles goodbye, thanks to MEAT EXTENDERS!" And that would probably sell $100 million worth of product, because late-night infomercials somehow caused both the Slanket and the Snuggie to move about a zillion units (TWO products where the business plan is "It's a blanket with sleeves—money, please!"). But meat extenders are something entirely different.

"Meat extender" is a term for basically adding something of value to meat to make it healthier. And we know what you're going to say: meat is bad. And we don't disagree! Meat *is* bad. And we all want people to stop eating it. But we also know that for some people, this shit is hard. And for some people, going cold turkey just isn't an option. For people like this, they need something to get over the hump. And if using meat extenders is one method to help get people eventually off meat, or if it can help reduce the number of animals slaughtered and brutalized along the way, then let's do it!

First, let's define our terms a little bit. When people

hear "meat extenders," they think that means that we're talking about adding sawdust to ground beef to screw people out of a few bucks, and that's not what we're talking about. When we're talking adding bulk to meat, there are typically two categories of stuff we're referring to: meat fillers, and meat extenders. Meat fillers are usually ground cereal grains and starches added to meat, stuff without much nutritional content that can add some volume to a pack of ground beef. These are not so desirable, other than how they're able to displace some of the meat that would otherwise be in that pound of ground round.

Meat fillers really came into their own, at least as something that grabbed the national consciousness, in 2011, when Taco Bell came under fire for offering beef that wasn't 100 percent beef. Taco Bell claimed that their taco meat mixture was about 88 percent beef and 12 percent spices, but was eventually sued by an Alabama law firm claiming that, according to their tests, Taco Bell's meat was only about 35 percent beef and 65 percent fillers of some kind. Taco Bell insisted this was not the case, and that their 12 percent of nonbeef was salt, pepper, spices, and things like oats and sodium phosphates used to make the texture ideal. Taco Bell's position was that their meat fillers were added to help with color and flavor, but they made no promises that their "spices" were used to make the meat healthier.

And that's the differences between fillers and extenders.

Meat extenders are designed to actually improve the meat that they're extending. These might include soy flour, soy protein, or ground mushrooms, or a host of other things. A lot of these extenders are purchased by consumers specifically to be added to meat to make the meat more healthy and as a strategy to use less meat in the meal. After all, if you're using 10 percent soy flour in tacos, that's a tenth of a pound of meat you're *not* eating. Everything nonmeat that you can add is, theoretically, meat that you're also taking away. And anything that uses less meat is a good thing!

But it's not just helping to cut down on meat consumption—these extenders are also making food more healthy! Soy flour, for instance, is full of good protein, to the tune of about twenty-nine grams of protein per cup. It's also a great source for folate, vitamin K, riboflavin, potassium, and magnesium. Sweet potato granules can increase a person's intake of fiber, beta-carotene, and other vitamins and minerals. Adding vitamins and minerals to meat? Not bad!

This is what people are adding on their own, to cut down on the meat they eat and to make that meat healthier. But can you also imagine these extenders used at an institutional level? Let's picture that future.

Imagine a country in the middle of a health crisis, a place where obesity is an epidemic and health-care costs are through the roof. You don't even need to have a great imagination, because that scenario is playing out right now in our country! But can you imagine a future where corporations say, "You know what—time for a change"? And then someone up the chain says that if you're going to have ground beef and ground turkey, you're going to have to sell it with meat extenders? So for every pound of ground beef you buy, 25 or 50 percent of it must be composed of soy flour or ground mushrooms or soy protein or whole oats or dehydrated sweet potato granules or rice bran.

Now, again, we don't encourage people to buy meat and eat meat. But if you had extenders like this on a wide scale, you'd have a ton of benefit. People would be eating healthier, which helps them out. And people would be eating a lot less actual meat, which would mean that a lot fewer fucking cows and turkeys and chickens would be killed. That's a win we'd take.

Maybe it won't happen overnight, with supermarkets changing how they sell ground beef. But maybe it starts at the institutions, where prisons start including more meat extenders, which results in healthier inmates and decreased costs. Then public schools start requiring it in their cafeterias, and the obesity rate and diabetes rate among school children drops dramatically, and the costs go down. It could happen.

I mean, it's not like we stopped eating Taco Bell, right?

> **FUN FACT:** Taco Bell has been one of the vegan meccas of the world for a long time now. There are over seven thousand Taco Bell restaurants.

CLEAN MEAT!

Eating meat is wrong. We're vegans; we stand by that. Pretty simple, right?

Or is it?

What if you could eat meat, and not only would it be cruelty-free, but it would be death-free as well? Does it change the equation? We know what you're thinking: *Wait, what? What the fuck are you guys talking about? Did you go off the deep end?*

Right now, people aren't just butchering meat, they're *growing* it. Food scientists are taking animal cells, growing them in culture, and producing meat in the lab. So here's our question: Can you eat that meat and still be vegan?

"Spare us your hypotheticals!" you say. "Who gives a shit about what might or might not happen in a hundred years?" But that's the thing. This isn't just some theoretical science fiction. This shit is happening *right now*. They've already grown a fucking hamburger!

In 2013, Dutch scientist Mark Post held a press conference/culinary event/tasting when he unveiled an all-cultured hamburger. The cost of the burger, from cell to bun, was a mind-boggling $350,000 (funded by Google's Sergey Brin, an animal rights advocate). At that price, you'd expect that would come with fries. And maybe a town house.

How'd they do it? They grew twenty thousand muscle fibers from cow stem cells in culture over three months. These fibers were then removed from culture and jammed together to make a patty. And then grilled. No cows were killed in the production of this hamburger. No cows were caged, prodded, poked, stunned, or tortured for this patty. This burger also didn't have some of the worrisome by-products that traditional ground beef does. Creating the burger didn't create hundreds of pounds of methane, nor did it involve a lake of toxic feces. The land required was a lab, not five thousand acres of grazing fields. All points in the column of clean meat.

This wasn't the first time that scientists had grown and cooked man-made meat. In 2003, Oron Catts and Ionat Zurr debuted in Nantes a tiny "steak" that they had grown from frog stem cells, which they proceeded to marinate in calvados (an apple brandy) and fry in garlic and honey before eating it. The verdict? Some described it as tasting like "jellied fabric." So, not a resounding success.

Still, it was exactly those kinds of experiments that caused PETA to take up the cause. PETA! An organization not known for their encouragement of meaty pursuits.

And yet PETA was so impressed by the idea of shifting meat production away from the slaughterhouse and into the lab that they offered $1 million to the first company that brought lab-grown chicken meat to consumers by 2013. And even though PETA didn't have to pay up, it was clear that they considered clean meat to be acceptable, even desirable. Meat without cruelty was the way to go, and arguably the way of the future.

What could the future hold? According to an article in the *Daily Mail*, under ideal conditions, labs working on creating cultured meat could produce fifty thousand tons of meat from ten pork muscle cells in the span of two months.

And growing meat isn't the only thing that these innovators hope to do. They also hope to make *better* meat. Dr. Uma Valeti was a cardiologist living and practicing in Minnesota. He was, incidentally, a vegan, because he's six different kinds of awesome. He was doing his thing, unclogging arteries and cleaning out fat from hearts, and he thought that if the problem was fatty meat creating the blockages, then perhaps the solution wasn't to address the blockages, but to change the meat. If people ate meat that was engineered to be safer, then perhaps he could save lives.

> **TRAGIC, DEFINITELY NOT FUN, FACT:** In the United States, every year about 735,000 people have a heart attack.

By growing meat in culture, he would have greater control over what kind of cells he'd be working with. Researchers have suggested that culturing meat would allow scientists to add the beneficial omega-3 fatty acids. Valeti founded Memphis Meats to see if he could make delicious, healthy, cruelty-free meat.

His efforts eventually led to his creating the first cultured meatball in 2016. The greenhouse gas emissions created by Valeti's process were 90 percent less than what would have been produced through traditional meat-making technology (specifically cows). The results were that it tasted like . . . a meatball!

The big problem was cost. At this point, Memphis Meats can produce a pound of beef at a cost of about $18,000. So a Quarter Pounder would ring up at about $4,500. Still a little expensive for a hamburger. That said, Valeti predicts that in another decade or two, "A majority of meat sold in stores will be cultured." Just think about the first flat-screen televisions. Those suckers were going for like $20,000 at first. Now you can snag one for under $300.

What is a vegan to think about this?

We think it's awesome!

As we've said before, we didn't become vegans as a way to revel in our nonmeat purity, or feel superior to people who ate meat. We became vegans because we wanted to spare animals pain and death. And eating clean meat accomplishes that goal. If we're eating a steak that was grown in a lab, then creating that steak didn't cause the death of an animal. It also didn't contribute to global climate change, or toxic runoff, or deforestation for grazing land, or, potentially, heart disease or erectile dysfunction. Those are all good things! We'd be happy to try clean meat.

MASSIVE CHANGE HAS ARRIVED

Necessity, they say, is the mother of invention, and necessity will demand that we change the way we eat. Increasing populations and decreasing resources will force people to look to new food sources, new food technology, and new cultural attitudes about what is acceptable or not acceptable to eat.

That said, it seems impossible to envision a future where the consumption of meat by the slaughtering of animals will continue to grow at the same rate that the population itself grows. There are just too many factors that will slow that growth. If it takes two thousand gallons of water to create a single pound of beef, then droughts and pollution will force food producers into looking at new options. As living spaces become more and more confined, there will be less and less tolerance for devoting thousands of square miles to the production of beef, pork, and chicken.

Younger people, not so indoctrinated into the habits of earlier generations, will be the first to seek new and better ways to feed themselves. Some will reject the bacon made by ripping off a pig's genitals and slitting his throat and instead opt for bacon that's grown in a lab. It won't be a future of "I must have something inferior, because I can't have what I want," but will instead be "I can have exactly what I want, and what I want isn't the flesh of a dead animal." The future will be exciting, sometimes confusing, and it will ultimately be better than what we have now. Because that's the way that progress works. Just sit back and enjoy the ride.

CHAPTER 10

TOTAL VEGAN WORLD DOMINATION

SO LET'S SAY YOU'RE THERE. You're vegan. Now what? You made it this far, which can only mean one of two things.

1. You hate us but you're a masochist and derive pleasure from torturing yourself.
2. You're ready to align with your preexisting values and save the animals already.

After you begin exploring vegan eating, you will begin to feel different. And you will begin radiating joy and happiness. Inevitably, people will walk up to you and say things like, "Dude there's something different about you.

You look like you're ready to take over the world or something. Are you Superman?" And if you're a woman, they'll ask if you're Wonder Woman.

And you're going to have to start responding with, "Yes, I am. Now come. Run with me as we bring about total vegan world domination. There will be nothing left. Let's get it."

Normally, the person will pass out for a second because they can't believe Superman or Wonder Woman is actually talking to them. They will be overcome with a joy they can't explain. But when they wake up they will run with you. And one will become two. And two will become four. And before you know it, the world is exactly the way we all want it to be.

People are eating their fucking veggies and Beyond Meat Chicken-Free Strips and petting all of the animals, not just dogs and cats. They're also petting cows, pigs, and chickens. Maybe even some fish, too. And we will all live in harmony.

In all seriousness, this is where you really begin to feel the shift. But it's not only happening with you; the shift is spreading to others, like a virus (the good kind). You're bringing your compassion and you're putting it out there into the universe. And other people look over and see that. And they become all like, "Holy shit! That's awesome. I'm going to do that, too!"

But before spreading to others, the shift happens inside of you. As you begin to explore vegan eating, you begin to feel more at peace with yourself. It's almost as if you never realized it before, but there was something missing that you couldn't pinpoint.

For both of us, it was as if out of nowhere we began to feel we were living more in line with our true values.

Many new vegans report people asking them, "Holy shit, dude! What the fuck did you do to your skin? It looks amazing!" To which some of them reply, "Holy fuck! I haven't eaten any meat or dairy in six weeks. I wonder if that's why."

Some people are asked how their hair looks so amazing. And if you're like Matt, you ask yourself, "Holy shit! When was the last time I used my inhaler?" To which you respond, "Holy shit! Months!"

Now we're not saying that is for sure going to happen to you. These are just anecdotes that have happened over and over again.

THE TIMES, THEY ARE A-CHANGIN'

Our friend Paul Shapiro, former vice president of policy at the Humane Society of the United States and author of *Clean Meat*, often talks about the craziness of different issues actually being legitimate social debate in the past. Not too long in the past, slavery was one of those legitimate social debates. Should it be legal or not to own another human being?

In the early 1900s, it was a legitimate social debate in the United States about whether or not women should have the right to vote.

And until very recently it was a legitimate social debate about whether two people of the same gender should be allowed to marry each other.

In all of these issues, there were people debating on the wrong side. And they were just normal, everyday people arguing for what they passionately believed to be right. Imagine meeting a lawyer or a doctor and hearing him or her say, "Slavery is a good thing. We should vote to keep slavery." It's hard to imagine, right?

But that's how it was with all these issues. At one point there were doctors, lawyers, congressmen, and police officers all saying, "Yes, it should be legal to own another person." It's almost impossible to fathom that today. If any lawyer in the United States came out and said, "I think slavery should be legal," she would quickly lose all of her business and her reputation.

But at one point in time, that viewpoint wasn't seen as crazy. And earlier than that, there were many lawyers who disagreed with slavery, but were afraid to say so publicly out of fear of losing business. Think about that shit! That sounds straight-up insane.

Yeah, that's right. The world changes.

It starts out slow. But before you know it, the next generation is born and assumes that shit happened a thousand years ago, not realizing that it actually happened very recently.

But it hits a point where it changes fast! And that's where we are at now in regards to abusing and consuming animals as food. You look back even just ten or fifteen years ago and it was normal to live in a place where there were zero vegetarians. For many, even just looking back five years, it was still fairly normal.

> Decades from now we will no doubt look back on many practices that are commonplace today, such as the treatment of livestock animals, in disbelief.
> —John Mackey, CEO, Whole Foods (excerpt from his book, *Conscious Capitalism*)

THE TIPPING POINT AND THE LAW

But today, even if you live in the sticks, you probably have at least one friend or family member who's vegetarian. If you live in a city, you're more than likely friends with at least a handful of vegans and vegetarians. And if you live in a huge metropolis, then you are probably friends and acquaintants with numerous vegans and vegetarians.

If you look at just your own life, even if you had never

thought about vegan eating until reading this book, you're probably already eating less meat than you did just five or ten years ago. We're reaching the tipping point.

Just look at how laws are changing. It wasn't that long ago that people thought that animals were just property. As long as you owned them, you could do whatever you wanted to them, and that shit was A-okay. But no longer. One of the newest developments in the legal world is that it's getting harder and harder to confine pigs to tiny gestation crates and chickens to battery cages. Ten states have already banned gestation crates (Arizona, California, Colorado, Florida, Maine, Michigan, Ohio, Oregon, and Rhode Island). About half of these legal changes were made via ballot measure. That means that the law came from direct democracy, from people who demanded change, rather than from politicians. The change is coming, and it's coming directly from the people!

And not just American people! In 2014, Canada voted to ban gestation crates *across the whole country*! Even Manitoba, you ask? Hell yeah!

But pigs aren't the only beneficiary of these new attitudes about animals. You know what else is on the way out? Battery cages. You know, those tiny fucking torture devices that chickens are often confined in? Well, that shit's going to stop. Battery cages are now illegal in California and Michigan, and are being restricted or phased out in Ohio, Oregon, and Washington.

How about baby cows? They're getting some help, too. There are now eight states that ban the use of veal crates (Arizona, California, Colorado, Kentucky, Maine, Michigan, Ohio, and Rhode Island). Not only are people turning away in droves from the idea of eating some poor little baby cow, but it's becoming legally impossible for agribusiness to give the people what they *don't* want.

And it's not just a state-by-state thing. In 2016, the FBI altered its view of animal abuse by stating that cruelty to animals will now be considered a "crime against society." This is significant, since it acknowledges that animals are a part of our society, that causing an animal pain degrades us as a culture. With the law in place, the FBI (the FBI— the ones who brought down Al Capone!) will be able to collect and track data about abuses against animals throughout the country. Under this rule, animal abuse will now be a Class A felony.

NEW INTERESTS FROM THE SPECIAL INTERESTS

These laws, and the spirit behind them, are also affecting corporate policies relating to animals. You know who else has demanded an end to battery cages? The egg industry! Even the egg industry, who's financially invested in putting as many chickens as close together as possible, said, "Enough." In 2011, the Humane Society of the United States and the United Egg Producers (the egg lobby—Big

Egg, if you will) agreed to support federal legislation that would eliminate new construction of battery cages, insist that the new cages replacing them be at least twice as large, require environmental enrichments for the hens (like places to walk and nest), and a host of other things to improve the lives of these chickens.

It was an interest in improving the treatment of chickens that led to the creation of the 88% Campaign (chickens account for 88 percent of the farm animals killed for food in the United States). Some very dynamic and influential companies agreed to partner with the 88% Campaign, including Starbucks. In 2015, Starbucks revealed a host of new corporate policies, including the phasing out of gestation crates and battery cages, and curtailing the use of growth hormones and the irresponsible use of antibiotics. Other companies, like Compass Group and Aramark, also signed on to the campaign.

> **FUN FACT:** By 2016, there were over thirteen thousand Starbucks stores in the US. And according to us, 100 percent of people agree that Starbucks is one of the greatest companies in the world. If you don't like Starbucks, it probably means you're not a person. P.S. Thank you to Starbucks for inviting us into the HQ in 2017.

And it's not just chickens and eggs. Pork sellers also want to see improved conditions for pigs. In 2014, industry giant Smithfield Foods, the world's largest pork processor and pork producer, asked the rest of the pork industry to phase out gestation crates so that they would be completely gone by 2022. Why this unexpected stance from a pork seller? Because their customers spoke up! Smithfield noticed that more and more people were getting sickened by how the animals were treated. Rather than be labeled monsters for contributing to animal cruelty, they changed their tune.

Things are changing! And you can feel it. Understand it! But we need to make it happen.

VEGAN IDENTITY

Before reading this book there may have been a stereotype or two in your head about who eats vegan. But now you've realized that the normal people are the ones who eat vegan. And half the celebrities in existence either already are 100 percent vegan, eat vegan often, or are about to become vegan.

So you've just decided to begin taking steps more in that direction. But still, you might feel yourself being pulled to become that crazy, stereotypical zealot you initially thought of. You know, the one who posts a million animal slaughter videos to Facebook per day and tells all his friends and family they are murderers at the dinner table. Yes, we know your pain. We've been there.

And we're here to tell you it's totally normal to feel that way. You now understand that it's standard practice in the pork industry to confine a mother pig in a crate so small she can't even turn around for basically her entire life. That it's common in the chicken industry to slice off a chicken's beak with a red-hot blade and no anesthesia. Who wouldn't want to run around yelling?

But now think about what was going through your head yesterday before you learned all this. You need to try to mesh both worlds together. Yes, it's insane. But you still need to interact in society like a normal human being, especially if you want to have any sort of impact on your friends and family.

Yes, it's time to change the world! The size of the role you play is totally up to you. Some want to have a massive impact. Some just want to do a small part.

Either way, if you want to influence your friends and family in a positive way, you can't let your emotions control you.

So now that you have decided to begin eating vegan, there's another goal that maximizes your impact to stratospheric proportions: your influence on others.

The goal for every vegan is to have the people around them look at them and say, "Holy shit! I want to be like you." And everyone can do it. There is no arguing. There is no debating. There is only being awesome and inspiring.

If you love having enemies, stop reading right here.

Because pretty soon every enemy you have will become your friend. And on top of that they will be living exactly the way you want them to live.

The suffering the animals are enduring can be overwhelming at times. But remember, they're counting on you to be their best ambassador. You need to do this right. Here are a few basic tips to help you maneuver through it all.

Don't Bring It Up Every Chance You Get

Your goal isn't to just force the word "vegan" into every conversation you have, or to talk about animal suffering at every opportunity. Don't spend every minute of the day being a wet blanket or a buzzkill. Your goal is to inspire the people around you to change, not to be a nag. So be strategic about when you talk about shit.

A good basic strategy to start with is "don't bring it up until you're asked about it," at least in the beginning. People are open to learning new things, but they don't want to feel like they're being forced into anything, or that someone thinks they're a bad person.

Eating Vegan Is Normal. Present It That Way.

There was an interesting study performed by Wes Schultz, an associate professor of psychology at Cal State San

Marcos, which focused on recycling and "normalcy." The study (reported in the *San Diego Union Tribune*) found that people would recycle if they thought that it served their own interests. People could act in a way that benefitted others, but they tended to feel more incentivized if they thought they were addressing some need of their own first. And one surprising way that people saw to benefit themselves was to fit in more. To be normal.

Basically, if people thought that their neighbors were recycling, then they were much more likely to recycle themselves, mostly as a way to feel more accepted and included in their community. Recycling happens more often when people think that it's normal to do, and it's less prevalent when people think they're acting alone.

Interesting.

Well, guess what?

Eating vegan is normal. And people are going to be doing it more and more because they're going to be seeing their neighbors doing it more and more. Eating vegan is going to be like someone yawning—you see it happen to someone else, and the next thing you know, you're doing it, too!

This is the most important way to talk about vegan eating. Research has shown that people are more persuaded to change their behaviors when other people around them are doing it.

Yes, we all have our ethics. But at the end of the day,

the most important question that guides us is "What is everyone around me doing?" Yes, it's kind of messed up. But shit is complex. And it's reality. No need to get upset about it.

The awesome thing about this is that eating vegan isn't just acceptable anymore. It isn't just something that people tolerate as some weird, marginal thing. These days, being vegan is actually the cool thing to do. So this thing is easy to do. Point out all the celebrities and professional athletes going vegan. It's the trendy thing to do, like smartphones and not dying from tuberculosis.

Remain a Positive, Happy, Upbeat Vegan Warrior

Yes, scientific research backs this up. But do we really need science to tell us that people don't like being around negative pieces of shit?

Think about popular culture in America for a second. The music, the people, the TV shows.

Is it depressing? Or is it happy?

It's happy.

Katy Perry: Happy. And hugely popular. Death Cab for Cutie: Sad. And a more cult attraction. (Also, let's not forget about The Postal Service, a Death Cab side project Matt thinks is even better than Death Cab. No offense, Death Cab.) *The Big Bang Theory*: Happy. A big hit. *The Leftovers*: Dark and sad. A small, devoted following.

People want to be happy. And they want to be around happy and positive people.

So the animals are actually counting on you to be a positive, upbeat person. Because when you aren't, you won't influence the people around you. And when the people around you are not influenced by you, animals are tortured and killed. Phil learned that the hard way, screaming at people and calling women murderers for wearing fur. Did that change the world? Did that make her not want to wear fur? Nope, it just made people want to avoid Phil, and also made people think animal advocates were a bunch of psychos.

So when you think about those chickens having their throats cut, allow that to serve as a reminder that you need to smile if you want that to end.

Encourage Every Step, No Matter How Small

Oftentimes people will focus on criticizing the shit they don't like in others. This in turn causes the other person to just hate you. And it usually also causes the other person to not change in any way.

However, when you focus all your energy on encouraging even the smallest shit, you will find that a whole new world opens up. When a person is encouraged in something, it makes them want to do it again even more. And most of the time it makes them want to go further.

For example, if your friend tells you he ate a veggie dog two weeks ago and thought it was pretty good, flip out with excitement.

"Holy shit, dude! You're probably the most amazing person ever for eating that. That's fantastic!"

Many people will often feel the need to encourage a further step. And they are normally wrong for doing so. There may be a time and a place to encourage a further step. But it is usually not during the first conversation about the other person eating vegan food. And in all honesty, it may never come up. The person will be eating vegan 100 percent of the time on their own before you even get a chance to bring up going further.

Stay Focused on How Awesome the Average Person Is

We used to live under this delusion that a lot of us live under, that people are horrible and don't care about anything but themselves.

We're sorry, guys. It's a delusion. And it's not true. People are awesome. It may be slow, but we're constantly improving. Things get better and better year after year. And humans are always changing shit for the better. Sure, there may be the occasional time when we humans screw things up and take things back a bit. But as a whole, we learn, and we make things better. For every piece of shit that exists, there are fifty people who are completely awesome.

And we'll tell you right now, when you believe in the potential of another person to be awesome, they will be awesome. But the opposite is also true. When you expect someone to be a piece of shit, they will be a piece of shit as well.

Talk About How Easy It Is to Eat Vegan

You now know about all the restaurants that offer vegan options, all the meatless options available at grocery stores, and that you can be the laziest motherfucker in the world and still eat vegan.

Break that shit down for other people. And when you're eating at some random-ass place like Buffalo Wild Wings, order the veggie burger. Five minutes into the meal, people will realize and be like, "Holy shit! I totally forgot you're vegan." And that's because you can blend right the fuck in now with all the options available.

Talk About It in a Way That's Relatable to the Other Person

If you think eating vegan is some radical thing, you're wrong. Like we said before, it's normal. So keep your answer normal. Keep it simple and to the point.

"I saw a video that showed slaughterhouses and had no

idea" is a pretty easy answer. If you want to go a little bit further, here's a good script.

"I saw a video that showed how the animals are treated. It showed how they confine the animals in cages so small they can't turn around, are mutilated without painkillers, and brutally slaughtered. I had no idea that's where meat came from. I've always been opposed to animal abuse. So once I learned that, I couldn't support it anymore."

You don't need to go on some tirade talking about some crazy philosophy you have. Keep it simple and relatable.

Don't Compare What Is Happening to Farm Animals to the Holocaust or Slavery

We love animals. We want them protected. But drawing this comparison is offensive to a lot of people. You can get the point across without doing it.

Listen!

Even when you are 100 percent convinced the other person is wrong, listen to what they say. Oftentimes when we talk to someone, while they are speaking, we just stand there, waiting for them to finish so we can speak.

No matter what you're talking about, listen and understand where the other person is coming from. If you're

unable to understand, don't give up. You have to keep trying.

When you make an attempt to understand the person
you are talking to, they will feel it. And a few things will
happen:

- You may find out you are actually wrong.
- You will become better at inspiring the other person to
  your side, because you know exactly what you need to say.

You Don't Need to Know Every Single Thing

Keep it basic. Many times it's actually better to just say,
"I'm not sure."

When you get asked shit about health, you don't need
to know the ins and outs of everything. You can literally
just say something like, "I don't know. But I know that
loads of professional athletes are going vegan now. And
they seem pretty healthy."

And you can always, always, always bring it back to animal cruelty. "I don't know. But they confine the animals in
cages so small they can't turn around, mutilate them without painkillers, and brutally slaughter them. Sometimes
they slit their throats while fully conscious. And that's why
everyone is going vegan nowadays."

Remember that this movement isn't just about you,
about what you think is right or wrong. It's not even just
about the animals, and saving them from torture and

death. It's about the whole world. It's about creating a world we live in where there's more water to drink, more land to live on, more food to eat, and a climate that won't kill us all. Making the decision to eat vegan benefits everyone. It cuts down on greenhouse gases, it creates more land that we can use to make healthier food, and it doesn't produce giant lakes of feces that can poison entire communities. These are all good things.

And you know something else? Eating vegan promotes ideas that will help our culture and help all of society. It's good to care about other living things. It's a good thing to recognize how interconnected we all are, and that thinking less selfishly can contribute to people trying to help each other, can lead to people working toward solutions to problems outside of our own relatively small ones. Eating vegan is a kind of statement. And that statement isn't just "I want to be healthier because I want my butt to look nice" (though we hope it will), but more a statement that "I want everyone to be healthier. I want to reduce everyone's suffering." That's a good place to be.

So raise a glass and give yourself a toast. Revel in how you're going to be on the winning side of this moment in history. You're going to be spared that moment when your kids or grandkids are talking to their friends, and some of them say, "Yeah, my grandma used to eat cows, but old people did lots of crazy shit that they didn't understand was bad." Everyone feels weird about having that crazy uncle who says things like, "My principal used to beat me with a switch, and it made a man out of me. . . ." Don't be that guy down the road. Be better.

There's a quote from the Talmud: "Whoever saves a life, it is considered that he saved an entire world." That's some deep shit. But there's truth there. Thinking about others means thinking about the rest of the world. Saving the lives of animals means you're trying to save the entire world. Hemingway, in *For Whom the Bell Tolls*, wrote, "The world is a fine place, and worth fighting for."

We agree.

Fight for it.

Fight for the animals.

Fight for your friends.

Fight for the future.

You're going to be glad that you did. And you're going to have a hell of a lot of fun on the way.

Now have a shot of vodka. You've earned it.

ACKNOWLEDGMENTS

Marian Lizzi, for understanding and believing in our vision. We knew after our first phone call that we needed to work with you.

Peter McGuigan, for having our backs when different editors tried to sway us from our vision. You were always right there to let them know what the fuck was up, in a nice way. You're one of our favorite people.

Allison Janice, if you had not e-mailed us in early 2015 and said, "I think you have a book," this book probably wouldn't have been written for another five to ten years. Thank you for reaching out.

Aaron Karo, for being a mentor of sorts in the beginning of our book-writing process. That was definitely when we needed you most. You instantly "got us" in a way that no one else does.

Michael Shohl, we are so grateful for your expertise, insight, and patience in putting up with us along our journey of writing this book.

FURTHER READING

DELICIOUS VEGAN FOOD:

¡Salud! Vegan Mexican Cookbook: 150 Mouthwatering Recipes from Tamales to Churros by Eddie Garza (Rockridge Press, 2016)
Nom Yourself: Simple Vegan Cooking by Mary Mattern (Avery, 2015)
*Thug Kitchen: Eat Like You Give a F*ck* (Rodale Books, 2014)

RANDOM BOOKS WE BOTH LOVE:

Think and Grow Rich by Napoleon Hill (Ben Holden-Crowther, 2017)
Change of Heart: What Psychology Can Teach Us About Spreading Social Change by Nick Cooney (Lantern Books, 2011)
The 48 Laws of Power by Robert Greene (Penguin Books, 2000)
When I Stop Talking You'll Know I'm Dead: Useful Stories from a Persuasive Man by Jerry Weintraub (Twelve, 2011)

Titan: The Life of John D. Rockefeller by Ron Chernow (Vintage, 2004)

Shoe Dog: A Memoir by the Creator of Nike by Phil Knight (Scribner, 2016)

What Is the Bible?: How an Ancient Library of Poems, Letters, and Stories Can Transform the Way You Think and Feel About Everything by Rob Bell (HarperOne, 2017)

RANDOM BOOKS MATT LOVES:

Psycho-Cybernetics: The Classic Guide to a New Life by Maxwell Maltz (TarcherPerigee, 2016)

Elon Musk: Tesla, SpaceX, and the Quest for a Fantastic Future by Ashlee Vance (Ecco, 2017)

Conscious Capitalism: Liberating the Heroic Spirit of Business by John Mackey and Raj Sisodia (Harvard Business Review Press, 2014)

Awaken the Giant Within: How to Take Immediate Control of Your Mental, Emotional, Physical, and Financial Destiny by Tony Robbins (Free Press, 1992)

Power Broker: Robert Moses and the Fall of New York by Robert A. Caro (Vintage Books, 1975)

Onward: How Starbucks Fought for Its Life Without Losing Its Soul by Howard Schultz (Rodale Books, 2012)

RANDOM BOOKS PHIL LOVES:

What It Is Like to Go to War by Karl Marlantes (Grove Press, 2012)

Man's Search For Meaning by Viktor E. Frankl (Beacon Press, 2016)

Genghis Khan and the Making of the Modern World by Jack Weatherford (Broadway Books, 2005)

Undocumented: A Dominican Boy's Odyssey from a Homeless Shelter to the Ivy League by Dan-el Padilla Peralta (Penguin Books, 2016)

The Score Takes Care of Itself: My Philosophy of Leadership by Bill Walsh (Portfolio, 2010)

Outwitting the Devil: The Secret to Freedom and Success by Napoleon Hill (Sterling, 2012)

Peace Is Every Step: The Path of Mindfulness in Everyday Life by Thich Nhat Hanh (HarperOne, 2008)

The Fish That Ate the Whale: The Life and Times of America's Banana King by Rich Cohen (Picador, 2013)

The Fiery Trial: Abraham Lincoln and American Slavery by Eric Foner (Norton, 2011)

ABOUT THE AUTHORS

MATT LETTEN

Matt was once asked to sum his life up in one word. What was the word?

Transformation!

He was extremely unhealthy and a hundred pounds overweight until the age of twenty-one, when everything changed.

His life has been transformed in just about every way one can think of. His career, thus far, has been spent as a fitness coach and serial entrepreneur, having launched three successful gyms in the Midwest immediately after graduating from college. Matt's performance, strength, and health were transformed when he went vegan. All the while he's been traveling the world, and trying his best to suck all he can out of life.

Matt believes every one of his transformations, from physical to mental to spiritual, have been put in place to help him transcend from the depths to the mountains, so that he can help others do the same. Along with his brother, Phil, they are doing just that.

PHIL LETTEN

Phil didn't learn how to hold a basic conversation with another human being until he was twenty-two years old and had already graduated from college. He developed his social skills while living out of a car for four years advocating for farmed animals. He has completed nine nationwide tours on behalf of the country's leading animal advocacy organizations, organized close to two hundred demonstrations on behalf of Mercy For Animals, been interviewed by several hundred mainstream media outlets, and given presentations to colleges, festivals, and other forums. He now enjoys bringing about vegan world domination in a new way through Vegan Bros.